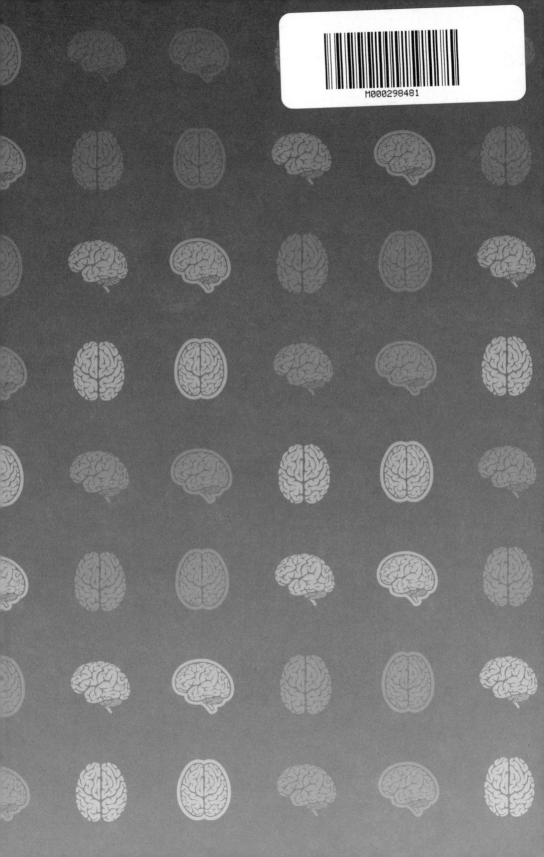

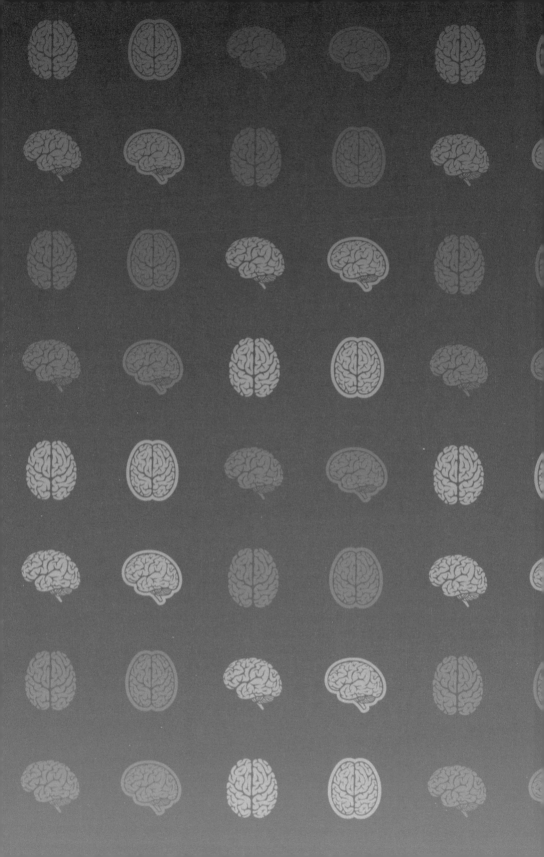

# TRUE LOVE

HOW TO USE SCIENCE
TO UNDERSTAND LOVE

FRED NOUR, MD

Published by

P. O. Box 6332
Laguna Niguel
CA 92677

ISBN: 978-0-9984043-9-4 (hardcover)
ISBN: 978-0-9984043-1-8 (softcover)
eISBN 978-0-9984043-0-1

Library of Congress Control Number: 2016919952

Cover design by © Fred Nour Graphics 2016
Interior designed by Mayfly Design and in the Minion Pro and Brandon Grotesque typefaces
Printed in USA
First Printing 2017

**Disclaimer**

While the publisher and the author have done their best efforts to prepare this book, they make no representations or warranties with respect to the accuracy or completeness of the information or the contents of this book. They disclaim any implied warranties of fitness for any particular purpose. No warranties may be created or extended by sales representatives or sales written materials. The advice and strategies contained herein may not be suitable for your situation. No content should be considered medical advice under any circumstances. You should consult with an appropriate, competent professional for personalized advice based on your own unique situation.

*To my daughters whose love inspired me to write this book.*
*To my wife who shares True Love with me.*
*To my patients who taught me so much about life, love, and courage.*

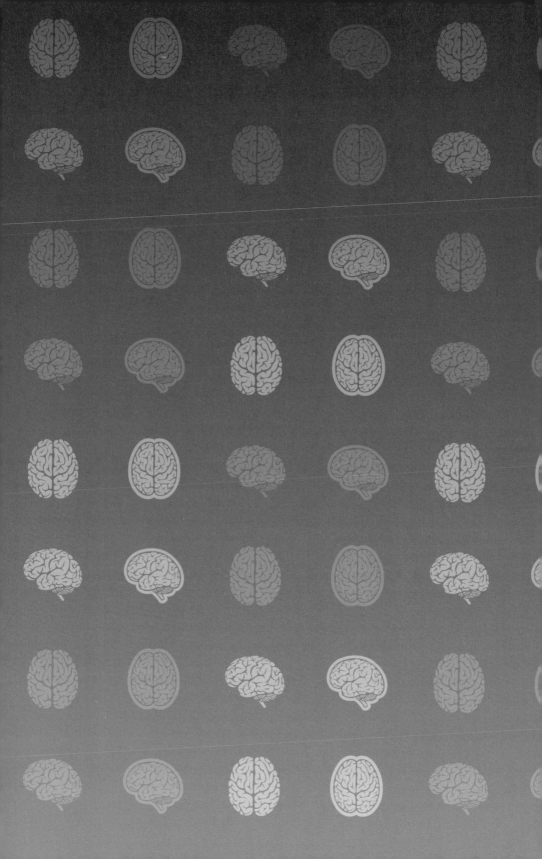

# CONTENTS

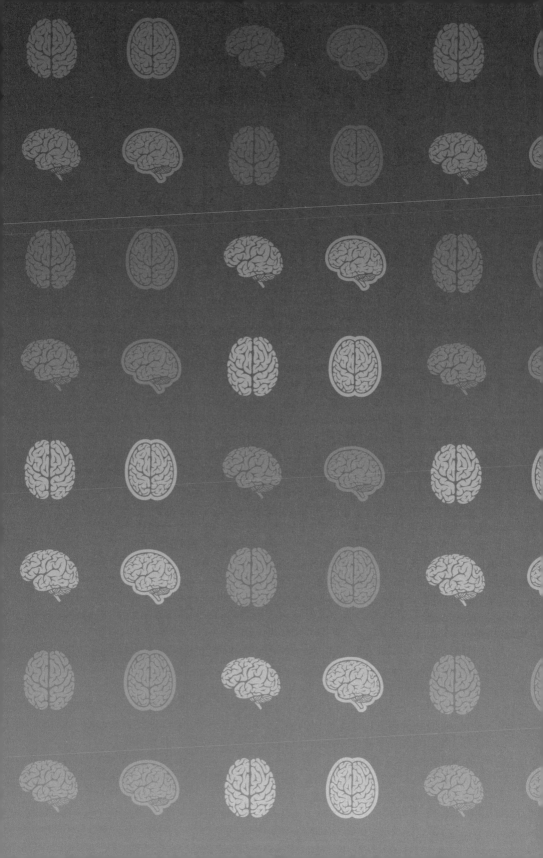

# ILLUSTRATIONS AND TABLES

*Figures*

## Tables

# FOREWORD

Everyone falls in love, and most of us do so more than once. Falling in love is innate and inevitable, and the process seems to be the same for all people in all places and all times. A 21st-century American in love knows exactly how the lovers feel in a love poem from China five thousand years ago. Or in love letters from India three thousand years ago. Or in the Middle East, in the Old Testament Song of Solomon from about one thousand years BC. We see love in Aztec pre-Columbian sculpture as well as Renoir's Impressionist paintings. Ethiopian nomads sang of love, and so did the Beatles; it is simply a part of being human.

It is also involuntary. Many languages, from French to Thai, affirm that we "fall in love." Love may not be undesirable, but it is unplanned, unpredictable, and uncontrollable. Our human intellect surpasses that of any other animals, yet there is something so fundamentally "built in" about love that when it happens to us, our rational thought is useless. We can neither wish love into existence nor will it to disappear.

Different cultures ascribe disparate explanations for the phenomenon of love. The ancient Greeks thought it was madness, and indeed, moping, mooning lovers can seem to be crazy, or at least irrational. Being pierced by Cupid's arrow would seem to be as good an explanation as any for why a love-struck man suddenly acts foolishly toward (clearly to others) an unsuitable woman. Other cultures have invoked bewitching, reincarnation, potions, Fate, and other machinations to account for the otherwise unaccountable emotion of love.

To a scientist, the explanation must indeed be rational and accountable. Any trait found in any member of a species must have a biological explanation. There is a biologic reason for anything so innate—so instinctive—and so universal. Yet until recently, love has resisted scientific analysis. It is provably difficult to study. How can we design a scientific experiment to analyze love? What can we measure? Does love, as the poets imply, come from the heart? Or rather, from a hormone?

Paradoxically, despite all we have said about love being irrational and unreasonable, it probably comes from the brain. Only recently have scientists developed experimental methodology and sophisticated technology to finally study love.

Does knowledge gained from scientific study destroy the wonder and beauty of love? Not at all. A rainbow remains resplendent and dazzling even after you learn it is only sunlight refracted off water vapor. Knowing how a magic trick is performed does not blunt its power but only makes it more astonishing when the observer is aware of the skill and practice required to produce the illusion. And even with the impressive details discovered about how the brain produces love, there will always be charms and mysteries of love we cannot penetrate. It will always be the most baffling of human emotions.

This delightful book, *True Love*, describes the fascinating studies that have solved many of the mysteries of love. These often complex and technical research studies are explained lucidly in layman's language while step by step, Fred Nour guides us through all the levels and layers of the brain, explaining how each facet of "love" has an anatomic and a biochemical basis. Drawing from biology, psychiatry, neurology, sociology, chemistry, and physics, Dr. Nour intelligently separates the scientific facts from unscientific fallacies. Nowhere else has this wealth of information been brought together in one single volume, and nowhere else has it been described so clearly. This book is a gem.

LOREN ROLAK, MD
Clinical Adjunct Professor of Neurology, University of Wisconsin
Adjunct Professor of Neurology, Baylor College of Medicine
Author of the internationally bestselling book *Neurology Secrets* (in
its fifth edition), *Neuro-Immunology for the Clinician* (in its second
edition), and *Coronary and Cerebral Vascular Disease: A Practical Guide
to Management of Patients with Atherosclerotic Vascular Disease of the
Heart and Brain*, as well as numerous medical journal articles

# PREFACE

Explaining love is a risky business.

Love is a strong emotion, after all, and pervasive among all humankind and many other species. Every woman, man, and child, from babyhood to adolescence, to adulthood and their final years, craves its wonderful feeling. No one can ever have enough of it, and I think it's safe to say we all want more love in our lives. All of us, whether conscious of this or not, are interested in maximizing our share of it.

Our share of love comes from our parents, our pets, our children, and others we hold dear, whether the "others" are people, or our beloved pets. We also share love with our mates, and this type of love is the topic of this book. Most likely, you decided to read this book because you want to maximize your joy from finding True Love and its lifelong happiness with a mate, either a current spouse or partner, or the one you hope to find.

To succeed in achieving this goal, this achieving of True Love, many turn to their friends and family or to advice books of various kinds. Worst-case, you might rely on unrealistic expectations based on what you've heard and seen in songs and movies while you were growing up. While I don't recommend the last option and will discuss the reasons why in this book, any or all of these sources might be helpful, or could actually be an impediment to your goal. I think you first need to understand what actually happens in your body, your mind, and your soul when you're in love. This core knowledge can help you direct your efforts and manage your expectations, so you can realistically attain your goal of maximizing True Love and its happiness. A large part of achieving this outcome happens in your brain.

Understanding those places and processes in the brain might just help you to find a mate, if you're looking for one, or to rethink and perhaps readjust your approach to a current relationship. In *True Love*, you'll find a comprehensible overview of what actually happens in your brain while seeking love, and well after. This knowledge should make your future decisions in any relationship more fruitful and rewarding.

Do you still remember your first love? Would it be fun to understand what actually happened in your brain that caused all those wonderful feelings?

Reading this book will help you answer some of life's seemingly unanswerable questions.

- What attracts us to certain individuals and not others?
- Why do so many of us marry the wrong partner?
- Why do so many people have difficulty finding the person of their dreams?
- Apart from joy and happiness, is there any purpose for love?
- Could love actually be a disease, or perhaps an addiction?
- Is there actual physical, scientific evidence for the chemical changes responsible for love, as some claim, or is that just a theory based on weak or false evidence?
- Are sex and love really the same?
- Do couples married for one year and couples married for twenty years share the same love?
- Is there anything we can do to grow our current love into the best and longest-lasting kind of love: True Love?
- Is falling out of love really "the end"?

Whether you're in a current relationship, looking for that special someone, or have had a relationship end and want to have insight into why it did, you'll find clues to the answers in *True Love*. And some of the answers you come up with by reading this book might surprise you!

So, how did I get to be an expert on True Love?

In the early 1990s, I was practicing in Chicago. As most neurologists do, I had many patients with multiple sclerosis, or MS, a neurological disease totally unrelated to love. My routine was to give each new patient an overview of the disease, and then explain how we would manage it together. Each presentation took about one hour. With three to four new patients per week, that meant three to four hours weekly doing the exact same thing. Seeking a more efficient way, one week I gathered all of that week's new MS patients into one room at the hospital and gave them the one-hour presentation, then allowed another thirty minutes for questions. Though I didn't foresee it, this was the beginning of a quite popular multiple sclerosis support group. Because MS strikes women more often than men, two-thirds of the members were women.

One day, the meeting fell on Valentine's Day, and some of the member-patients wanted to hear my thoughts on love. Since I had an interest in understanding the basis of love, having loved and succeeded, and also loved and failed, I decided to write a lecture entitled "The Neurology of Love." After presenting it to the group, comments were varied. Some thought the presentation was great, some thought it was okay, and some simply hated it. One attendee even said, "I don't like it. You killed the mystique of love." Despite such mixed reviews, each year the group's leaders asked for the same lecture, near Valentine's Day. I modified and improved the lecture each year, incorporating more discoveries relating to our understanding of love.

Some stayed in the group but avoided the annual Valentine's Day lecture. Most of the romantics didn't care for the "love lecture," so they never came back for the annual love lecture. Realists mostly liked it, and returned with more questions.

With a successful series of lectures, you might be asking, "Why did he decide, after all these years, to write this book, and why now?"

My two daughters are reaching their late teens and soon will start to look for love, marriage, and family. Recently, I tried to open up a discussion with them about love. Tried to, that is. "Dad, you're from an ancient culture," one said. The other explained, "We're a new generation. Everything we think or do is totally new and alien to you. Why waste your time and ours to talk about ancient beliefs about love?"

Later, musing on their reactions, I thought, *Maybe if I write my knowledge and experience in a book and many people find it useful, they'll reconsider my ancient beliefs and read the book!*

Or, perhaps not. But I continue to believe a science-based learning approach to the *why* and *how* of love will benefit many in need of the knowledge. In my practice and via extensive research, I've found a few things that help in achieving true, lasting love. I want to introduce these to those who need this help. Yet today, I keep meeting people in their fifties and sixties who never married because they, to paraphrase, "haven't yet met the person of their dreams." Perhaps their difficulty was partly caused by the fantasy fairy tales they learned and believed in as children. Indeed, I hope *True Love* will stimulate a public debate about the effect of media directed toward children and young adults on the formation of unrealistic expectations for a mate later in life. Maybe public discussion can lead to changes in how these fantasies are presented to children. I also see people who divorce three and four times, each marriage ending because the couple "fell out of love." Each one of these marriages had children, and those children are at high risk of being disillusioned in their own marriages. It's my hope that this book helps many couples avoid this unfortunate cycle.

An additional goal of this book is to improve the accuracy of the available reading on this topic. In this era of plentiful and popular self-help articles and books, many people have learned about the science behind love from lectures, books, media interviews, and newspaper articles. Most were written or given by authors in related fields, and some of these authors included incorrect medical facts in their books. There are many ways to study the brain, which I will outline near the end of this book. However, the great majority of these nonmedical authors' writings were based on only one way to look at the brain, the fMRI (functional magnetic resonance imaging) scan, a test that has drawn recent, serious concerns about accuracy.

In fact, the summer of 2016, as I wrote *True Love*, was the climax in the debate that fMRI images could be fallacies. The most respected *Proceedings of the National Academy of Sciences* journal, in its July 2016 issue that contained a study about fMRI, reported that over 70 percent of images seen on fMRIs are false positives, based on the most extensive review of fMRI data by a group of Swedish and British scientists. The National Academy of Science published a request to recall many of the forty thousand articles based on fMRI! No less than the American Association for the Advancement of Science published the following report in its prestigious journal, *Science*: "Brain scans (fMRI) are prone to false positives, study says. Common software settings may have skewed the statistics for thousands of studies" (*Science*, July 15, 2016). The Massachusetts Institute of Technology (MIT), with the University of California San Diego, published an article titled, "Puzzlingly High Correlations in fMRI Studies of Emotions, Personality and Social Cognition," questioning the statistical methods used by some.

To put it simply, these associations and publications are considered the gold standard in the field of scientific research, and I don't make such assertions lightly. And now, many people who've watched and read and listened to all the hype about pictures of "the brain in love," pictures of "the love center" in the brain, and so on, are understandably confused about what is fiction and what is fact about our knowledge of the neuroscience of love. So, one goal of *True Love* is to correct these factual inaccuracies for you, the reader, by sorting fact from fiction. Even more, I hope my attempt at correction will help steer future research on love in the right direction. To these ends, I've included an appendix with an in-depth section about the recently discovered problems with fMRI.

Most of what you'll find in *True Love*, however, is drawn from my experience with real human beings, including my experiences in my neurology practice, yet I researched and used outside sources. Most of the studies used in *True Love* were of heterosexual couples. The same general principles governed my writing about love among homosexuals, with differences in studies noted where they occur. Many pieces of our knowledge about emotions came from animal studies, which I acknowledge can be controversial, but the information gained from these studies is of great value. So, in forming this book to make it as helpful and comprehensive as possible, I drew from information based on animal research, chemical studies, genetics studies, and also clinical data—put most simply, clinical data are facts drawn from human behavioral responses to changes in brain chemicals from drugs used to treat certain brain diseases.

Most of what you'll read in *True Love* is based on scientific facts that are all but proven by many scientific studies. However, some gaps exist and are filled in by me, based on my theories and the theories of others. At this time, we don't have the technology to fill in some missing pieces in our knowledge about love. Fortunately, as science continues to advance, we'll find other, better technologies to help us better understand our brains and, consequently, ourselves. For now, for some aspects of love, we can only presume what happens while waiting for the final, definitive proof. I wrote facts in close-ended sentences, for example: "Every culture believes in love." Theories are mentioned using qualifying words such as, "most likely," "probably," "I estimate it to be," and so on.

Throughout the book, to help make the complex simpler to understand, I've used song lyrics, mostly of popular songs I personally like. The eloquence of these lyrics is beyond my composition talents. Perhaps there are other songs and poems you like better. If you do, please let me know via the book's website, www.truelovebook.net.

I've made a great effort to make brain science as simple as possible, though sometimes this is hard because our brain systems are complex. To enjoy the book fully, I've included sections for those wanting to understand some basic concepts about how our body works. If you find those parts boring, then skip them; you'll still enjoy the reading.

While *True Love* is a great beginning, I want to make this book, eventually, an all-encompassing source for understanding love from all its angles as perceived by the great majority of people. Love is so enormous, you see, that it can't really be written about by just one person. I'll have blogs on the book's website to explain in more detail about different aspects of studying the brain in love, and an email feature on the site for your feedback. I welcome hearing your feelings and thoughts.

Whether you're a romantic who's satisfied with your current beliefs about love or a realist who's more interested in "insider information" that can help you make love better and long-lasting, my hope is that you find what you seek within the following pages. And I very much look forward to your feedback about love at www.truelovebook.net.

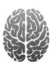

## CHAPTER 1

# THE WHERE AND WHEN OF LOVE

Perhaps it's more accurate to say, where in the world do people believe in love?

Love is a truly universal emotion, and is reported in all cultures and throughout known history. No culture disavows or disbelieves in love. Dr. William Jankowiak looked at love in 186 of today's cultures. Previous to his work there was a belief that "romantic love is a European contribution to world culture." Dr. Jankowiak and his group found evidence for love in 88.5 percent of cultures that had left folkloric (oral) stories or written materials about love. What about the other 11.5 percent, which left no written or oral record? These didn't leave evidence for love, yet there was no evidence that these cultures *didn't* believe in love. The scientists also found that even the people of the extremely isolated Kalahari Desert in Africa believed in not one, but two types of love. One was described as "rich, warm, and secure," as seen in a spouse's love. The other love, associated with a lover, was termed as "passionate, exciting, but often fleeting and undependable."

Were there always two types of love, as believed in the most primitive culture in Africa? Is that still true today?

Or, are my daughters right to say, "We're a new generation. Everything we think or do is totally new and alien to you. Why waste your time and ours to talk about ancient beliefs about love?"

*Has* love changed over the centuries? Do our feelings today differ a lot from the very old days? Let's see what history tells us.

Love is probably 150 million years old, per scientific research.

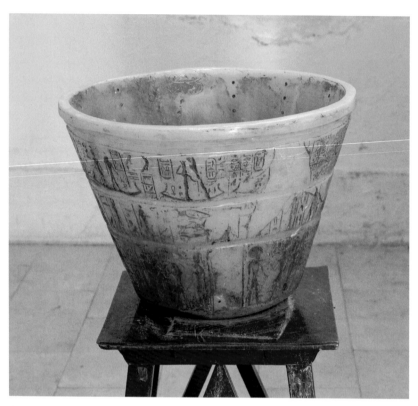

*Ancient Egyptian vase*

Current research tells us love probably exists in different formats in more primitive species, but in past research, as it is now, we can only find evidence for love or sex in late vertebrates (animals with a backbone), which includes humans.

It seems the Egyptians wrote the earliest recorded human love songs, romantic poems with lyrics intended to be sung aloud. Scant evidence for but no proof of this form of expression exists prior to this era. Love songs were engraved on the "Cairo Vase," which Egyptologists estimate to be from the 19th or 20th dynasty of the Pharaohs. This estimation dates the vase to between 1,300 to 900 BC, about three thousand years before today.

To give you a feeling of how love was perceived three thousand years ago, I'll give you one song from this vase. You can compare these lyrics to how you feel about love today, and decide if love has changed over the past three hundred decades.

A few notes first: The words "brother" and "sister" in the songs don't refer to siblings, but are terms of endearment. Brackets [ ] indicate words added to allow for better understanding of the song. Words on the vase too faded to interpret are replaced with a (?). Parentheses ( ) are used to explain some words.

Now let's enter the world of the poet who wrote the songs, and see how one poet told the love story of one boy and one girl three thousand years ago.

(Girl)
*[I think] of you day and night*
*when I'm lying down and when I wake [up] in the morning*
*[I am] Just thinking of (?)*
*your voice [awakens] desire*
*that makes my body feel alive*

*When I grow tired [of waiting]*
*I remind myself (?)*
*"There is no one else*
*to balance his heart. Only me."*

*Your love is as lovely*
*as oil and honey [to the throat],*
*as fine clothes to nobles,*
*as clean robes to the God's bodies,*
*as fragrant incense to the nose*
*of a worshipper coming in [the temple from the street],*
*[as a signet ring] to a finger.*
*Love is like dates mixed with beer;*
*it's like [wine] [mixed] with bread.*

*We will be together,*
*even beyond the grave.*
*I will be with you each day.*
*This woman's one wish fulfilled*
*a life spent serving her lord [her lover].*

*As the north wind blows*
*I so enjoy going down to [the Nile]*
*I would love to go down there*
*and bathe in front of you*

*So you could see how nice I look*
*in my tunic of royal linen,*
*shining with oil,*
*my hair plaited with reeds.*
*I'll go down to the water*
*and catch a red fish*
*that just fits in my hand.*
*I offer it to you*
*while you admire my beauty*
*O my brother, my hero,*
*Please [come] see me!*

Now stop and ask yourself: Does this poem, dated millennia ago, sound like the love feelings we have today? Did the feelings change over all those centuries?

Next, let's look at the boy's feelings.

(Boy)
*There she is right in front of me.*
*My sister is coming to me*
*My heart dances and I open my arms to her.*
*My heart is at home like a fish in its holding tank*
*O night, be mine forever,*
*now that my queen has come!*

*When I hold her*
*I am transported to Paradise.*
*Then it's like the (?)-plant*
*crushed into an ointment*
*She is fragrant like perfume.*
*We kiss, lips parted*
*Who needs beer?*
*My emptiness is filled,*

*Sekhmet's (Egyptian Goddess of curses) claim annulled.*
*As she leads me to her bedroom,*
*Come [servant],*
*Put fine linen under her when you are preparing her bed,*
*See to it that you use the good white linens.*
*The surface of her legs*

*seems drenched in fine oil.*

Now stop and ask yourself: Does the boy's response sound like the romantic feelings we have today? Did the feelings change over all those centuries?

Other poems or songs on the vase describe similar feelings, so it wasn't just *this* girl and *this* boy who held such deep feelings for each other. Since this couple wasn't the only one with such deep feelings for each other, now let's look at the oldest-known written love poem, just to see if the feelings are different in that one.

The earliest written love poem in history, that I know of, is much older than the

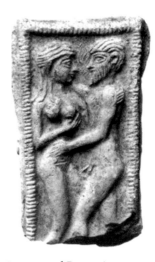

*Inanna and Dumuzi*

ones found on the Cairo Vase. This one came from Mesopotamia (present-day Iraq) about four thousand years ago. "The Love Story of Inanna and Dumuzi" was celebrated in Mesopotamia in a big festival held annually and became so important and famous that this is probably the origin of our modern-day Valentine's Day celebrations.

Though I shortened the poem significantly, it's still a bit long, but I wanted you to *feel* the passions of love four millennia ago.

There are five characters in this poem:

- The goddess Inanna (meaning "the great from above," also referred to as Venus)
- Her brother, the sungod Utu
- The shepherdgod Dumuzi
- The farmergod Enkimdu
- Inanna's mother Ningal
- (A few other goddesses are mentioned casually.)

## The First Time Inanna Meets Dumuzi

Inanna meets her brother Utu in the fields.

Utu tells her that the fields look beautiful. The flax (plant used to make white sheets and dresses back then) looks lovely. He can use it to make her a beautiful wedding gown because there is a suitor for her.

Inanna feels scared and tries to convince him it's too complicated to make the dress and the sheets. It's much easier to just cancel the whole thing and relax. Utu assures her he will take care of everything and that she need not worry.

When Utu tells her that the new suitor is the shepherd Dumuzi, she rejects that. Let's read and *sense* the feelings and thoughts as perceived by Inanna.

Inanna:
*Nay, the man of my heart is he*
*Who has won my heart is he*
*The one who hoes,*
*His grain storehouses are heaped high,*
*The grain is brought regularly into the storehouse,*
*The farmer, Enkimdu, he whose grain that fills all the grain storehouse.*

Utu:
*Sister of mine, marry the shepherd,*
*His cream is good, his milk is good,*
*The shepherd, whatsoever he touches, is bright.*
*His good cream he will eat with you,*
*He, the king protector,*
*Inanna, marry the shepherd*
*Why are you unwilling?*

Inanna:
*I and the shepherd will not marry,*
*I will not wear his coarse garments,*
*I will not accept his coarse wool,*
*I, the maid, the farmer I will marry,*
*The farmer who grows many plants,*
*The farmer who grows much grain.*

Dumuzi appears in the fields and hears what she said. This so infuriates Dumuzi that he speaks out vehemently in his own defense with the repeated claim that he has much more to offer than the farmer.

Dumuzi Replies

*The farmer more than I! The farmer more than I!*
*The farmer, what has he more than I?*
*If he gives you his black flour,*
*I give him, the farmer, my black sheep,*
*If he gives me his white flour,*
*I give him, the farmer, my white sheep,*
*If he pours me his prime beer,*
*I pour him, the farmer, my yellow milk*
*More than I, the farmer, what has he more than I!*

Inanna isn't impressed. She still has concerns.

The goddess Inanna has misgivings about his pedigree that, she claims, is quite inferior to her own. It's only after Dumuzi demonstrates that his pedigree is as good as hers that she consents to go out with him on a date.

Dumuzi is so happy she will go out with him on a date, as the poem states:

*Dumuzi rejoiced, he rejoiced,*
*On the "breast" of the river he rejoiced,*
*On the riverbank, the shepherd, on the riverbank he rejoiced.*

## The First Date

Inanna meets Dumuzi in the fields. Dumuzi tries to embrace her.

She tries to free herself from his embrace. Since she does not know what to tell her mother, Inanna pleads with her lover:

*Come now, wild bull, set me free, I must go home,*
*Dumuzi, set me free, I must go home,*
*What can I say to my mother Ningal!*

But her lover has an answer that Inanna, noted for deceitfulness, was only too happy to hear from his lips:

*Let me inform you, let me inform you,*
*Inanna, most deceitful of women, let me inform you,*
*Say my girlfriend took me with her to the public square,*
*There she entertained me with music and dancing,*

*Her chant the sweet song she sang for me,*
*In sweet rejoicing I was lured and the time passed.*
*Thus deceitfully stand up to your mother,*
*While we by the moonlight indulge in our passion,*
*I will prepare for you a bed that is pure, sweet, and noble,*
*I will spend time, the sweet time, with you in plenty and joy.*

## After the First Date

Inanna sings on her way home:

*Last night, as I, the Queen of Heaven, was shining bright, was dancing about,*
*Was uttering a chant at the brightening of the oncoming light,*
*He met me, he met me,*
*The lord Dumuzi met me,*
*The lord put his hand into my hand, Dumuzi embraced me.*

## A Marriage Proposal

Dumuzi must have proposed to her, since the goddess is singing exultingly and ecstatically on her way home:

*I have come to my mother's gate, in joy I walk,*
*He will sprinkle cypress oil on the ground,*
*To my mother he will say the word,*
*To my mother Ningal he will say the word,*
*He whose dwelling is fragrant,*
*Whose word brings deep joy.*
*My lord is respectfully asking for the holy groin.*

## Wedding Daydreams

*When for the wild bull, for the lord, I shall have bathed,*
*When for the shepherd Dumuzi I shall have bathed,*
*When with (?)[1] ointment on my sides, I shall have adorned,*
*When with amber (reddish paste), my mouth I shall have coated,*
*When with black on my eyes, I shall have them painted,*

---

1. To remind: (?) means faded word on the clay tablet.

*When, in his fair hands, my loins (hips) shall have been shaped,*
*When the lord, the shepherd Dumuzi, lying by holy Inanna,*
*With milk and cream the groin shall have smoothed,*
*When on my vulva, his hand he shall have laid,*
*When on the bed he shall have caressed me,*
*Then shall I caress my lord, a sweet fate I will decree for him,*
*I will caress Dumuzi, the faithful shepherd, a sweet fate I will decree for him,*
*I will caress his loins; the shepherd-ship of the land I will decree as his fate.*

## The Marital Promises

Inanna tells Dumuzi that she will always be supportive of him:

*In battle I am your leader, in combat I am your armor bearer,*
*In the assembly I am your advocate,*
*On the campaign I am your inspiration.*
*You, the chosen shepherd of the holy shrine (?),*
*You are the king, the faithful provider for Inanna,*
*In all ways you are fit*
*To hold high your head on the lofty dais [2][raised platform], you are fit,*
*To sit on the lapis lazuli [Sapphire] throne, you are fit,*
*To cover your head with the crown, you are fit,*
*To wear long garments on your body, you are fit,*
*To wrap yourself in the garment of kingship, you are fit,*
*To carry the baton and the weapon, you are fit,*
*To guide straight the long bow and the arrow, you are fit,*
*To fasten the throw-stick and the sling at the side, you are fit,*
*For the holy scepter in your hand, you are fit,*
*For the holy sandals on your feet, you are fit,*
*You, the sprinter, to race on the road, you are fit,*
*To jump on my holy bosom like a lapis lazuli [Sapphire], you are fit,*
*May your beloved heart be for the longest of days.*
*What (highest god) has "An" (goddess of sky) determined for you, may it not be altered,*
*Enlil, the grantor of fate—may it not be changed,*
*Inanna holds you dear, you are the beloved of Ningal (Inanna's mother).*

---

2. Again, [ ] means words added to explain meaning.

## The Official Business: Dumuzi Goes to Her House to Propose

The shepherd Dumuzi comes to Inanna's house, milk and cream dripping from his hands and sides, and clamors for admittance.

After consultation with her mother, Inanna bathes and anoints herself, puts on her queenly robes, adorns herself with precious stones, and opens the door for her groom-to-be. He asks her parents' permission to marry her.

Inanna exalts Dumuzi after his official proposal:

> *I cast my eye over all the people*
> *I called Dumuzi to the godship of the land,*
> *Dumuzi, the beloved of Enlil,*
> *My mother holds him ever dear,*
> *My father exalts him.*

## The Wedding Night

> *She bathes, scours herself with soap,*
> *dresses in her special "garments of power,"*
> *She has Dumuzi brought to her prayer-and-song-filled house and shrine*
> *to sit happily by her side.*
> *In the house of life, the house of her father the king,*
> *Inanna dwelt with him in joy.*
> *"Plow my vulva, man of my heart!*
> *"Me, the Queen, who will station his ox there?"*

She later moves to Dumuzi's kingdom to live in his house.

## Marital Life

Once happily settled in the king Dumuzi's house, the goddess utters a plea and makes a promise. The plea is for milk and cheese from Dumuzi's sheepfold:

> *Wild bull, Dumuzi, make yellow the milk for me, my bridegroom,*
> *I will drink fresh milk with you,*
> *The milk of the goat, make flow in the sheepfold for me,*
> *With (?) cheese fill my holy churn*
> *Lord Dumuzi, I will drink fresh milk with you.*

And her promise is to preserve her spouse's "holy stall," which seems to be a symbolic designation of the king's palace:

*My husband, the godly storehouse, the holy stall,*
*I, Inanna, will preserve your house for you,*
*I will watch over your "house of life."*
*The radiant wonder place of the land,*
*The house where the fate of all the lands is decreed,*
*Where people and (all) living things are guided,*
*I, Inanna, will preserve it for you,*
*I will watch over your "house of life,"*
*The "house of life," the storehouse of long life, I, Inanna will preserve for you.*

Let's stop here and try to analyze this love poem as it would have been perceived at the time it was written.

- Is this a love story, or not?
- Did Inanna truly love the farmer, and was she persuaded by her brother to marry the shepherd, Dumuzi, instead?
- How can we tell if she really loved the farmer?
- The shepherd went from being nobody initially to being "a bull." What actually happened in her body, mind, or soul to cause her to change her perception of him? If she fell in love with the shepherd, is there any behavioral evidence that she fell in love with him?
- Inanna talks a lot about the physical attraction: about sex. Did she fall in love with Dumuzi, or did she merely have lust for him?

- Is this a story about sexual love, romantic love, True Love, or just a routine love?
- Is sexual desire the first part of love?
- Is love only about sex?
- Is sex-equals-love just a male bias toward females?
- Are sex and love not related to each other at all?

Returning to our original question, has love really changed by much in the last four thousand years? I don't think so, and likely, you don't either. More to the point: love has been around a long, long time, so there must be some purpose for it to have lasted so long.

What *is* the purpose of love?

Or, as Tina Turner asked, what's love got to do with it?

- Is the perception of love just to induce joy or happiness in us?
- Is it a trick played on our minds by our genes to get us to breed, and so preserve the species?
- Is it to get us to select the best mate to improve our genes, and thus improve our species?
- Is it to keep a couple together until they have offspring that are old enough to survive?

•  •  •

So: is there any physical, scientific evidence for a link between sex and love?

There is so much to analyze and discuss about this old story. You and I will gradually answer all these questions later on, as we discuss the different phases of love and their effect on us. By doing this, we'll understand how all this happened to Inanna, and in the process, we'll understand more about ourselves.

CHAPTER 2

# OVERVIEW OF LOVE

## Defining What to Some Can't Be Defined

When I described explaining love as risky business earlier, I wasn't joking—it's difficult for anyone to explain love to someone else, and when the subject is love, emotions tend to run high. Besides, we all have our own perceptions of love, even when the love isn't real. Think about a book you read that was later made into a movie. Some people might feel the book was much better than the movie. Why is that? After all, a novel is a story, and the movie relays the same story (or at least, most of the same story). So why would anyone love the book, but feel let down by the movie, or vice versa?

Reading is an active experience, in that you are involved in taking those "words on paper" and crafting images of them in your mind. The movie is the book as perceived by the director and the actors; the images and even the sounds are created for you. A movie will never fully match the images you created in your mind while you read the book.

It's the same when you read a book about love. What a writer defines as "love" might not reflect or exactly match *your* view of love.

Another risk of explaining love is that we, as a culture, seem entranced by the *mystique* of love, the mystery of love. A person attending one of my lectures once told me, "It (love) is *magic* that just lands on us from heaven." We don't want to believe that real, physical changes in our brain cause these wonderful feelings. We want to believe that there is magic in it and that it is not merely a switch in our brain flipping on or off.

Another example of the risk in explaining love can be found on your television. When you see a movie like *Titanic*, full of action, emotions, beautiful music, and dramatic, well-acted scenes, you feel, however temporarily, that these are real people. It's hard to believe that the effect on you is based on electronics. Hearing that from me, you might feel that the magic of TV has vanished, or become just another boring flow of electrons. You might feel disappointed by what I just revealed.

If you prefer the fantasy rather than the reality about love, you might be happier reading love stories, listening to love songs, admiring love poems, or listening to beautiful music inspired by the creator's perceptions of love. This will match your dreams about love, and perhaps you'll be satisfied with that.

For most of us, the choice is that we either try to understand love or simply give in to the mystique of love. Understanding love's nuts and bolts—how love works—might well make it easier to achieve the perfect love you've dreamed about.

So, each of us has our own concept of love, as do I. Here is my definition of love:

Love is a person's *subjective feeling*, which produces a subjective sense of joy, excitement, and happiness. This feeling is *derived from* a relationship with one specific human being. That feeling induces a *motivation* for specific, love-induced *behaviors*. The *behaviors* associated with love are unconsciously oriented toward the preservation and improvement of our species.

That feeling of love is hard to put into words that will satisfy everybody, but we all know it, from previous experiences with love from a very young age. It's good that each of us has our own, unique experiences to draw from, because no words ever existed that truly describe the unique *feeling* of love. It's like tasting a certain kind of cheese. You'll immediately recognize the cheese when you taste it again, but describing the feeling associated with it (the taste) to someone else isn't easily put to words.

In summary, love is:

Feeling ➔ Joy ➔ Motivation ➔ Certain Behavior ➔ Improvement and Preservation of Our Species.

Now we have a better idea of what love means to you and me, but the question from earlier remains. What's love got to do with it? In this case, "it" is the improvement and preservation of our species.

## Why Do We Need Love?

When I lived in a house by a lake in suburban Chicago, I watched the Canada geese reproduce on the lake's island. Geese lay two to nine eggs each spring. In four weeks those eggs hatch, and goslings emerge. The goslings come out of the eggshell and *immediately* can walk, swim, and feed themselves. In another six to eight weeks, they're able to fly and live independently. By the next spring, each former gosling takes up a mate and is ready to lay eggs and have its own goslings.

In only one year, the life cycle repeats itself with another two to nine young goslings.

If we compare that to humans, it takes us nine months for (usually) only one egg to hatch (deliver) into a baby, a baby that is, in effect, born prematurely. Due to the progressive increase in the size of the brain over time, the baby's head became too big to go through the bones of the birth canal, so it has to be delivered earlier than full physical maturity. Even so, full brain maturity takes about eighteen years. That "prematurely" born baby (after nine months of pregnancy) is unable to care for itself, can't feed itself, can't walk, can't talk, and certainly can't swim like a newly hatched gosling can. It takes many years until that human baby can be self-sufficient, and perhaps as long as fifteen years before that baby can have its own babies.

Compared to geese and most other species, this is an exceedingly slow life cycle.

Because of this, humans needed a unique system, one that would get the parents to stay attracted and bonded to each other for a long enough time so the young child would be protected and nurtured to near reproductive age and full maturity. Love is there to achieve that goal. Yes, love. Our brain evolved that system when we developed a new part in the brain called the *intermediate limbic brain*. We'll learn more about the intermediate limbic brain in the next chapter. For now, it's enough to know that our genes carry special codes to ensure that love will happen, and that these genes guide the manufacturing of certain chemical "products" in our brain. These chemical products convince us that the mate we're with is just perfect, even if he or she isn't. Not a flawless system, then, but on the upside, these chemicals make us feel that our bond will last forever and that any problems will be easily overcome. These chemicals also make us feel that it's also a joy and total pleasure to be with that specific person. Even more, they produce a strong urge in our mind that tells us we must.

*Fall in love and have a family* isn't simply a worried parent speaking. This strong urge or desire isn't conscious or voluntary, either. But the effect of these gene codes tends not to last forever. Fortunately, nature developed a fix for that problem too. Later on, another set of chemical products in our brain bonds us more strongly together. These chemicals induce a good, long-lasting feeling: True Love. This feeling should last us a lifetime.

So you might already be asking, what are these chemicals? Or perhaps, if love is located in our brain, then how do these chemicals affect our brain to almost *force* us to love and have a family?

Next I'll give an overview of the biology behind love. After that, you'll find more details about the phases of love.

## The Biology of Love Basics

Scientific research tells us there are two main brain-chemical systems. Medically speaking, these chemicals are the *neurotransmitters* involved in love. These chemicals are monoamines and nonapeptides. All behaviors that we think of as love-related are based on the effects of these two chemical systems on the brain.

The monoamines family includes catecholamines (dopamine, epinephrine, and norepinephrine) and serotonin. These are the "reward chemicals," but the effect is associated with other feelings as well; for our purposes here, monoamines are responsible for the "falling-in-love" or "romantic" phase of love. We'll talk more about monoamines in a later chapter, because they have a lot to do with the falling-in-love phase of love. Monoamines affect the early phase of love, the one that shows up in that heady rush of feeling makes our pulse race and our minds refuse to allow us to fall asleep even though it's way past bedtime.

Nonapeptides, namely oxytocin and vasopressin, are the chemical substances responsible for the feeling of permanent love, or what I call the True Love phase. I'll leave it there for now, but you'll learn a great deal more about these chemicals in later chapters, when we'll be discussing the all-important True Love phase of love. We might say that learning how to achieve True Love is worth the wait!

For now, it's enough to know that while nonapeptides are the main players in this "game of true love," there are other chemicals you'll see as you read along, which includes the names of sex hormones responsible for sexual behavior. Sex isn't love, but sex helps enhance love; also, it's love that stimulates sexual behavior.

Many other neurotransmitters are involved too, but I'll minimize their discussions to keep things simpler.

All that's for later. Now I want you to know about the stages of love.

## The Phases of Love

Grown-up love, to the surprise of some, is like the wonderful experience of having and loving a child. Both these important life events happen in four phases.

### First Phase

In having a child, a woman prepares to get pregnant by being sexually developed and physiologically (physically) mature, and it takes many years to achieve full maturity.

In love, this phase is the dreaming of "the Person of My Dreams"—the mate selection phase. This phase doesn't suddenly happen when a person becomes an adult, or sexually mature, however. It starts in childhood and continues until we meet that person and immediately "fall in love." Yes, you prepare for love from a very young age, from the time children are playing with dolls and learning to admire and even developing a crush on their preschool teachers or a classmate or two.

### Second Phase

In this phase, a woman (and a man, of course) performs the act of getting pregnant and carrying the baby to full term. There is intense joy and pleasure with the conception, followed by the phase when the mother experiences the wonderful awareness that she's carrying a fetus that will mature to be her beloved child forever.

In love, this is the "falling-in-love" or "romantic love" phase. Chemically speaking, this is the monoamines phase of love, because there's some scientific evidence that this phase happens by a well-orchestrated, large increase in catecholamine effects in the part of the brain I mentioned before, the intermediate limbic brain, and coordinated by serotonin. These excess monoamine effects usually last for about two years, and this is the phase we in science believe to be the "love" or "romantic love" phase. When monoamine ceases its increased effects, we move on to the next phase, falling out of love. If you're feeling panic at what you just read, please don't despair that falling in love lasts only two years. There's so much more to love than that!

### Third Phase

In having a child, a woman goes through delivery. It's miserable and painful. She hates it. It's necessary, however, to have the desired permanent baby she wanted so badly.

In love, this is the falling-out-of-love phase. This phase happens when the monoamine effects are reduced to their usual, normal level, and not enough nonapeptides have been released to sustain the loving feeling. We're no longer in romantic love. We fell out of love. But, there is another type of love on its way.

### Fourth and Last Phase

In having a child, the woman has the baby in her hands and is enjoying nurturing and loving it for a lifetime, even as the stages of childhood maturity (and need I say, adolescence?) create necessary separations. Once a mother, always a mother, it's often said, no matter how much time, distance, or angst has or might occur between the mother and her child.

In love, this is the phase where if you've hung in there, past the initial bloom of romantic love, past the depths of falling out of love, you'll be experiencing true, lasting love. Chemically speaking, this is where the nonapeptides have kicked in and induced lifelong love. This is the love experienced by couples who've been married for five to ten years or more. This phase is chemically powerful, and permanent. This is True Love.

. . .

To understand how all these chemicals work to create such sweeping and life-changing effects, I'd like you to know some basic information about the brain chemicals and how they work. Actually, it's a good idea to back up a bit more, for a brief look at how our brain cells communicate. Next, we'll compare how the brain structures in animals correlate to their behaviors. This will help us understand how and where love alters our human perceptions. Skip it if you wish and continue with the rest of the book, but I think you'll benefit from knowing.

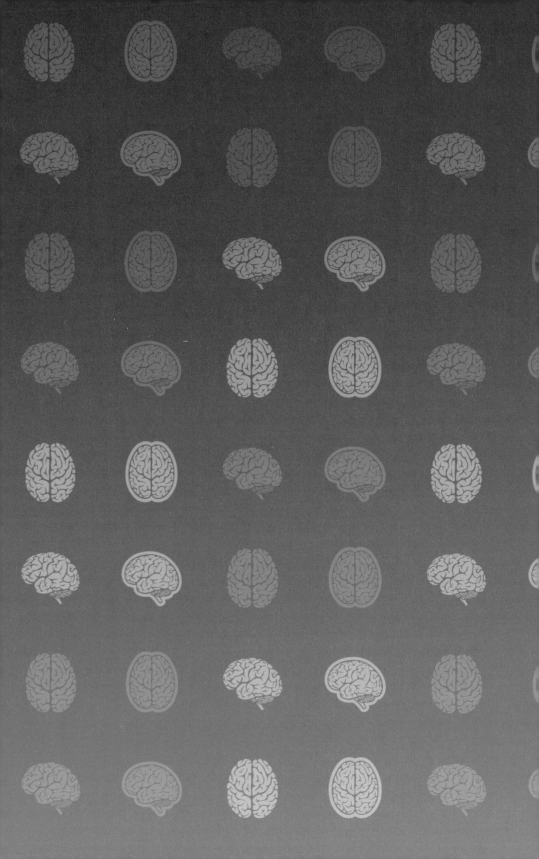

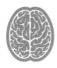

CHAPTER 3

# BRAIN FUNCTION IN A NUTSHELL

As scientists, we know that crocodiles and frogs (reptiles) don't know love. We also know that birds do know love. In fact, we know that some species of birds pair up for life. By comparing the crocodile's brain structures to the brain structures of the bird, we can find the parts of the brain responsible for love. If we then compare the brains of birds to the brain structures of humans, we can understand how we feel love differently from birds and reptiles, and why.

So let's take a look at how the brain structure changed between species, and how the new structures brought about by those changes affect our behaviors.

The brain basically has three parts.

This short table shows the brain's main functions, and is a simplified way to look at the parts of the brain. In reality, it's more complex than this. Even so, this view is enough to understand what we're interested in right now: love and its underlying chemicals.

Now let's talk about these three brain parts in more detail.

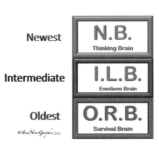

Basic brain parts

## Old Reptilian Brain: Our Survival Brain

*(illustrated in red)*

This is the oldest and most primitive form of brain, and I call this brain part the *old reptilian brain* because it's seen in reptiles. The typical reptile-family members with this brain structure include snakes, turtles, crocodiles, lizards, and frogs.

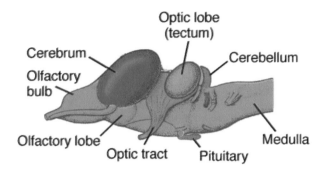

*Frog's brain*

The old reptilian brain is the biggest part of the frog's brain. It promotes *survival* by making the heart beat and the lungs breathe, and organizes swallowing actions to get us to eat.

The frog's brain possesses a very small *new brain* (in blue) to make survival decisions: *Should I jump now, or wait?* There is a tiny intermediate limbic brain (in green) that sits just above the pituitary gland. This is composed of one part only, called the *hypothalamus*, which is responsible for the sex drive.

Based on this brain structure, reptiles (crocodiles and frogs) can survive, think a bit, and know sex at a rudimentary level. Here's a bit more to help you become more familiar with these functions and how they make the old reptilian brain different.

**Survival**: The old reptilian brain has a primitive defense system for protection. For example, this brain has quick reflexes that compel the reptile to jump away from nearby threats. I'm sure you've seen a frog make one strong, big jump back into the pond. The famous "knee jerk" we experience during neurological medical examination uses this reflex. When a doctor taps on your knees or other limb parts, he's checking your old reptilian brain functions.

As a neurologist, I've seen many patients with only the old reptilian brain surviving, the rest of the brain damaged from traumatic injuries or lack of oxygen, or other serious disorders. We call this a "chronic vegetative state." A person can survive with their basic functions of the heart beating, automatic breathing and swallowing, and a stable blood pressure, but that person can't feel any emotions, can't think, and can't do anything specific at will, such as moving any part of the body because they want to. A person can live for many years with just the survival brain, the old reptilian brain.

**Reproduction**: Sex evolved a long time before love came along. The sex drive emerged about five hundred million years ago with the development of the Chordata (the early vertebrates), which includes fish species. The fish brain has a part developed to control the sex drive, the hypothalamus. Reptiles reproduce by laying large numbers of unfertilized eggs. They have sex acts for fertilizing the eggs but don't protect their offspring and have nothing to do with them after laying the eggs. If they see another animal destroying their eggs, they couldn't care less and don't move or react at all. If they happen to still be around when their eggs hatch, they're disinterested and detached from their offspring. This is because reptiles have no intermediate limbic brain. Reptiles know sex, since they have a hypothalamus, but don't know love.

**Love**: Actually, the lack of ability to love is the hallmark of old reptilian brains. Reptiles don't affiliate (bond) with a specific mate and don't raise or protect their offspring. We know that frogs make a mate selection for the period of reproduction, but then each mate goes his/her own way.

When I compare the brains of birds and humans a bit later on, you'll notice that the structure of the old reptilian brain doesn't change in the more advanced species, even in humans. We still inherit mostly the same structure and functions of the old reptilian brain, just as DOS software in the 1980s was the same DOS system used in many subsequent Windows versions. DOS software stayed the same while Windows software evolved further with time.

## Intermediate Limbic Brain: Our Emotion Brain

*(illustrated in green )*

The next phase in our brain structure was the development of the intermediate limbic brain. Typical animal members with large old reptilian brains *and* large intermediate limbic brains are birds and penguins. And of course humans. (Soon, we'll get to what makes our brain so different from that of other animals.)

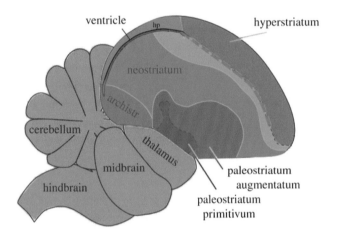

*Bird's brain*

The avian (bird) brain preserves the same structure and function of the old reptilian brain (red). The bird can survive with this old part of the brain, but notice the addition of a new, large brain part (green). This is the intermediate limbic brain. Birds have a small new brain (blue) to make decisions such as *Should I fly higher or lower to avoid this attacking bird?* (We'll be learning a lot about the new brain next. For now, just know that the new brain is a more advanced brain.)

This intermediate limbic brain (green) part sits on top of the old reptilian brain. Looking at the brain from the outside, the intermediate limbic brain is visually separate from the third phase in brain development, the new brain (illustrated in blue colors), which is quite convoluted in humans (for a reason you'll find out later) but not in birds. In fact, the intermediate limbic brain's name came from the word "*limbus,*" meaning "well demarcated" from the human's new, convoluted brain.

What makes the intermediate limbic brain unique is that it has a sort of master control room. In the US Defense Department, there is a "central command center" that coordinates the activities of the various military forces: the Air Force, the Navy, and so on. The intermediate limbic brain has such a center: the hypothalamus.

This new, huge intermediate brain part introduces emotions in our brain, as well as many improvements in our functioning. Since this is the brain part responsible for most love-related emotions, I'll spend more time describing its functions and effects as related to love. I'll still describe its other functions but with fewer details.

The intermediate limbic brain improved our reproduction success by improving the mate-selection process. It improved our ability to protect ourselves as well. Its addition to the old reptilian brain introduced reward systems, which motivated us to seek love, as we'll explore later on. It introduced memory systems so we could save our experiences with other mates and remember our joyful experience when we're in romantic love. It improved our adaptation to the environment and improved our body awareness and control, which changes our perceptions when we're in romantic love.

## Improved Reproduction through Olfactory System (Sense of Smell) Development

It might seem odd, but it's true; the ability to discern scent was the first special sense to evolve in animals. It started to develop in fish and continued to advance. There are two such systems: a main scenting system and an accessory scenting system. The accessory scenting system is involved in socio-sexual functions. With this accessory system, the animal can tell various odors of mates and foes apart. The animal can recognize its mate, its offspring, its friends, or its enemies. It's used for mate selection and mate identification. After the sex center in the hypothalamus, the accessory scenting system is probably the second-oldest center in the intermediate limbic brain.

With the development of vision and hearing, the importance of odor identification declined. The skull became crowded with big eyes and a large hearing system. The ability to detect and distinguish various odors started to decline as animal brains developed further. Dogs smell things humans can't. However, the ability of the accessory scenting system continued its social behavioral importance. Dogs must still sniff people to decide who they are. And we humans still do this, though we do it unconsciously. Animals and humans developed sense-making organs, predominantly in the armpits, so scents can and are used for mate selection and identification.

Look at this picture of what most would call a sexy woman. She has her arms up on her head and is showing you her underarms. She appears to do this unconsciously, so unless those advising her on her pose are aware of the "scent system"

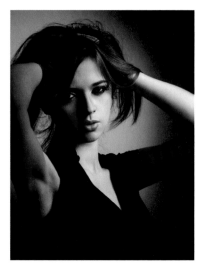

*Smell and attraction*

just described—unlikely—she probably isn't aware that her unconscious move is one millions of years in the making, designed so a male can smell her scent (via chemicals released called *pheromones*) and select her as his mate. In return, the mate perceives her as sexy, also without being aware of why he does. This is because the intermediate limbic brain functions unconsciously, without our awareness.

I've seen the effect of scent on emotions in my practice. A woman came in with symptoms of depression. Her husband was an engineer. His job duties included selecting suppliers of parts from China, which required him to visit China, perhaps a month or more at a time. Quite understandably, she missed him and felt depressed when he was gone. A challenge was that she was so sensitive to antidepressants that those weren't a good option for her. I recommended that she try saving his pillowcase, his bedsheets, and his towels from the laundry, and that she should smell them whenever he was away. She came back impressed, saying that not only did she not miss her husband to the degree of getting depressed, but also that she was surprised that the "dirty clothes" actually made her feel happy and that the clothes smelled "so good."

I recall meeting a woman on a date in my youth. When I came close to her to say good night and give her a hug, I noticed that she smelled bad. I asked my friend, who'd known her well for many years, about her body odor. To my surprise, he said he didn't smell anything unusual, except for the woman's nice perfume, which I didn't detect at all. Our next date, remembering what my friend had said, I tried to pick up on that "nice perfume," but to me, she still smelled repulsive. She was otherwise a wonderful girl, but I had to stop seeing her. Later on, I'll reveal why I consciously rejected her smell when others couldn't perceive any odor problem at all. (Hint: it's in our genes.) In fact, when I later talk about the effect of our genes on our mate selection, you'll see more evidence for the important component of smell in mate selections in humans.

## Improved Reproduction through Emotional Interest in the Offspring

For reproduction to be successful, one must have live offspring that remain alive for as long as possible—at least long enough to be independent—and ideally long enough for they themselves to reproduce. The chance of that first goal, independence, went up with the addition of the intermediate limbic brain, because it added emotional interest in offspring, which means the animal defends, rears, and protects its offspring. Parents bond together to share the rearing of their offspring, and they risk their lives to protect their young one. Reptiles, who lack an intermediate limbic brain, will do absolutely nothing about you taking a few of their eggs away. Try to take an egg from a Canada goose nest and see what the parents will do to stop you!

## Improved Reproduction through Improved Mate Selection

An elaborate system evolves for selecting a mate, a process aimed at improving the species by improving the gene selection. I'll say no more about this here. It's best if this is discussed when we talk about mate selection in the first phases of love, in a spot where we'll have plenty more room.

## Improved Protection through Fear

Fear is an important function of the intermediate limbic brain that can be lifesaving. Fear helps improve animal survival better than the old reptilian brain can. If the animal with an intermediate limbic brain perceives a threat to its life, as perceived by any of its senses such as seeing, smelling, or hearing another predator, it will immediately feel fear.

The intermediate limbic brain fear center developed connections downward to the old reptilian brain, to improve the response to the threat. Fear sends downward signals to the old reptilian brain that makes the heart beat faster and the tubes in the lungs open wider to allow more oxygen into the blood. It diverts blood away from the digestive system to the more important organs, the brain and muscles. Who wants to eat if you feel you're about to die?

With this new intermediate limbic brain, the animal in fear can run faster and farther away from the threat or bite the predator harder and so on. With fear, the chances of survival are much better than the simple jumping reflex of the frog. The fight-or-flight response starts to evolve.

## Improved Protection through the Autonomic Nervous System

There is a new connection from the intermediate limbic brain nervous system-to-old reptilian brain nervous system called the *autonomic nervous system*. "Autonomic" means "automatic." The furnace in your house turns on automatically when the thermostat senses that it's too cold. It shuts off automatically when the thermostat senses it's warm enough now. This is an automatic system. The furnace belongs to the old reptilian brain; the thermostat belongs to the intermediate limbic brain of the house. The thermostat (intermediate limbic brain) tells the furnace (old reptilian brain) when to act and when to cease to act.

This autonomic nervous system has two components. One component makes things run faster—the *sympathetic nervous system*—and one component—the *parasympathetic nervous system*—slows things down. This works just like the acceleration and braking in a car that makes driving easier, more balanced, and safer.

When we see our beloved, our heart beats faster and stronger, and we sweat, all because of the increase in brain activity in the catecholamine family of chemicals. This increase in brain activity causes our sympathetic nervous system to increase its functioning (firing rate). Catecholamines include the chemicals dopamine, norepinephrine, and epinephrine. A strong emotion, such as fear, activates the intermediate limbic brain, which then activates the sympathetic nervous system. To be more specific, norepinephrine nerve connections cause the heart to beat faster and stronger; this is perceived as palpitations.[3] Norepinephrine also causes an increase in sweating. Epinephrine causes the sense of fear.

## Improved Behavior through the Introduction of Reward Systems

The intermediate limbic brain system offers plenty of protections, as mentioned above, and also some upsides. The following "joys" act as rewards that motivate us to seek more love and love-related behaviors.

### Joy in Play

An animal with an intermediate limbic brain discovers the joy from playing as well as from doing certain behaviors. Look at the dog fetching the ball back to his owner so the owner can throw it away again, for the dog to catch the ball again and again. The dog isn't interested in the ball itself. It's the game that gives the dog a sense of joy, from catching the ball. That joy is perceived in the intermediate limbic brain. This joy is scientifically proven to be from the release of dopamine in the intermediate limbic brain system. Two lovers feel extreme joy from playing games together.

### Joy in Eating

Eating causes us a sense of joy. Think of the wonderful feeling you had eating that delicious meal at that fancy restaurant, or at home, cooked by your gourmet spouse. Food stimulates the same "lust center" in the intermediate limbic brain that sex and play stimulate. We all love and crave chocolates because chocolates are proven to stimulate the same lust center.

### Joy in Social Behavior

Socialization is part of this intermediate limbic brain system. The intermediate limbic brain organizes social behavior and our relationship with members of our community. We feel joy by just talking to other people and exchanging ideas, views, and feelings. We feel more joy when we're around people than when we're alone. Our joy of being with that special loved one comes from this. Conversely, we punish criminals by depriving them of the ability to socialize. We place them in jails or, even worse, in solitary confinement.

---

3. Palpitations are the conscious awareness of heartbeats.

### Joy from Addictions/Compulsions (Drugs, Gambling, and so on)

Okay, this one might not be such an upside, but the intermediate limbic brain is the system involved in drug addictions. As an example, cocaine releases monoamines in the intermediate limbic brain. Monoamines cause a sense of joy. Once the reward is learned by the intermediate limbic brain, the urge (motivation) to do drugs again and again becomes powerful and irresistible. Gambling and compulsive shopping follow the same mechanism.

### Joy of Sex

Scientists easily proved that the sex drive is dependent on the level of sex hormones in the blood. If you give male animals more androgen (testosterone), their sex drive increases. If you give female animals more sex hormones, their sex drive will also increase. This happens from the effect of these hormones on the hypothalamus in the intermediate limbic brain, not from their effects on any other part of the body. We'll discuss sex drive more later on, but for now, it's enough to know that the intermediate limbic brain reward system strongly motivates us to seek more rewards. Sex acts and orgasm release dopamine in the intermediate limbic brain, and that causes a strong sense of joy. The intermediate limbic brain "learns" the joy, and seeks it again and again. Similar to all intermediate limbic brain functions, this behavior isn't under our voluntary conscious control.

### Joy in Happiness

Joy, happiness, rapture, ecstasy, bliss, elation, euphoria, exhilaration, pleasure, and rhapsody are words lovers usually use to describe their feelings when they're in romantic love. Whatever word might be chosen to describe the feeling, a sense of joy, contentment, and happiness is associated with activity in the intermediate limbic brain. In addition to the catecholamine release, love causes the release of serotonin, a brain chemical, which makes us feel relaxed.

Once this feeling is "learned" by our intermediate limbic brain, it motivates us to seek the same sources of the joy and relaxation repeatedly, and urgently. An everyday example: the elaborate schemes some people design in order to have sex with a certain individual for the joy of sex and the sense of relaxation afterward. Significant motivation to seek a reward! All of these joys came from the intermediate limbic brain and didn't exist in the old reptilian brain.

## Improved Mate Selection through the Introduction of Memory

When we have the one we wanted to find, it's great and fine. When we search and search for where we put those missing keys or that last container of yogurt we're just certain we saw in the back of the refrigerator, the subject of memory isn't our favorite. Memory is complex to discuss, because our memory uses complex brain systems and involves two brain parts: the intermediate limbic brain and the new brain.

The intermediate limbic brain does its part by inducing a strong encoding of all our memories. The more emotions associated with an event, the more likely its memory will last forever, or however long "forever" actually lasts.

Almost everybody will recall the purchase of his or her first car. I certainly do: memories of being in the showroom, who was with me, which make, color, and model I purchased. Of course I was quite excited about having my first car ever. After that I bought many other cars but don't recall the details nearly as well as I recall that first car with all its tagged-on emotions. Actually, I have no memory of some cars I bought in the past, but that first car purchase remains clear in my memory.

Be it thirty or forty or even more years ago, we all remember our first kiss in very fine detail: the when, where, and how things went at that remote time. Yet, can you recall if, on September 18, 2016, you had kissed or not? September 18, 2016 is much closer to today, but unless you have the rare disorder hyperthymesia, which actress Marilu Henner has been reported to possess, you have absolutely no recall.

Yes, we all have selective memories. The memory recall depends on the emotions associated with the event rather than the event itself.

Other memories are stored in the new brain, but those are saved for a much shorter period. On a vacation, I recall staying at a particular hotel. The room number was useful when I was a guest at the hotel. Once my vacation ended, I totally and permanently forgot my room number. Can I now recall my room number at that hotel? I can't, because the room number had no emotional impact on me and has no importance now.

Strokes affecting the new brain aren't associated with significant memory loss, but as a neurologist, I see cases of people who experienced strokes affecting the intermediate limbic brain memory centers. Their memories are totally and permanently erased, and these patients have great trouble remembering anything, whether recent or remote.

Speaking of memory, here is what's important to remember here: new brain memory is short-lived. Intermediate limbic brain memory, due to the retention power of emotional impact, is potent and exceedingly permanent. It isn't erased as easily as the new brain memory. Later, we'll discuss the use of memory in mate selection.

## Improved Adaptation to the Environment through Circadian Rhythm

Does our love behavior change between nighttime and daytime?

The word *circadian* came from *circa* (around) and *dies* (day). *Circadian rhythm* is the name for our twenty-four-hour internal clock. This is seen in humans and animals, and also in plants, fungi, and some bacteria (Cyanobacteria). An example in plants is the flower petals that are closed at sunrise, wide open by noon, and closed again by sunset.

Many bodily functions are controlled by the circadian rhythm: our body temperature, thirst, and fluid balance. That maestro of the intermediate limbic brain I mentioned earlier, the hypothalamus, controls our circadian rhythm.

## Improved Adaptation to the Environment through the Hormonal System

The intermediate limbic brain also has influence over the *hormonal system*. The intermediate limbic brain can increase or decrease the amounts of hormones that are released. Again, we have no conscious control over the release of hormones, but the intermediate limbic brain does.

This is probably how the emotion of love stimulates the desire for sex with one's beloved at night more than during the day. The intermediate limbic brain releases more sex hormones, and the hormones act on the intermediate limbic brain, causing sex acts–desiring behavior. The sex acts cause a release of dopamine. Dopamine release in the intermediate limbic brain causes the joy of sex that is perceived. That joy motivates the intermediate limbic brain to ask for more sex. The animal doesn't know why it wants the sex but knows that doing so creates a sense of joy.

I recall watching a documentary about fish reproduction. It showed a male fish looking right and left continuously to locate fish eggs. Once it did, it dove down to fertilize the eggs, then moved on with its search for more eggs to fertilize. Imagine that I can talk to that fish. If I asked the male fish, "Why do you keep doing this?" I expect him to say, "I don't know why. I only know that doing so makes me happy somehow." The fish has a small hypothalamus for having sex, but no other intermediate limbic brain parts to cause love for another fish. The fish has merely become obsessed about sex due to the chemicals released in the intermediate limbic brain system and wants it released again and again. This isn't love but merely joy from an act.

## Improved Adaptation to the Environment through Sleep

Sleep is controlled by the circadian rhythm, a part of the intermediate limbic brain. Why do we need to waste one-third of our lives sleeping?

The simple answer is that without sleep, we die. It's true that when we fall in love, we become sleepless due to the effect of the catecholamine norepinephrine on the sleep center. Thankfully, the sleeplessness that can occur with falling in love doesn't bring such a dire consequence.

## Improved Adaptation to the Environment through Fatigue

We feel rested after a good night's sleep. A bad night's sleep leaves us tired, fatigued. If we have emotional turmoil, we feel fatigued, with usually no desire to do anything. We call this feeling "emotionally drained." (This is probably serotonin related.) Fatigue is an intermediate limbic brain function that triggers us to find the cause of our fatigue, and often, the solution is to simply get more rest.

## Improved Adaptation to the Environment through Our Feeding Cycle (Hunger and Satiety)

Hunger gets us to eat. Satiety gets us to stop eating. The intermediate limbic brain controls both, as a toggle switch controls the overhead lights in most homes. This ability probably evolved to adjust to the variation in food supply from seasonal weather changes. Interestingly, the intermediate limbic brain center that controls hunger and satiety is the same center that controls sexual desire. It makes us feel that we want to have sex or don't want it at all. However, there is no satiety center for love.

## Improved Adaptation to the Environment through Stress

*Cortisol,* also known as "the stress hormone," is also controlled by circadian rhythm. Stress affects our processing of emotions; it's difficult to feel too passionate when we're stressed. (For simplicity, we won't get into how cortisol interacts with our brain chemicals.)

## Improved Adaptation to the Environment through Improved Cell Functions

This is unrelated to love, so I will skip it.

## Improvement of Body Awareness through Improved Sensations

This section most definitely relates to love, especially concerning sensations and special sensations.

All our special sensations are connected to the old reptilian brain and from there to the intermediate limbic brain. Smell, vision, touch, taste, hearing, and balance/movement are all eventually connected to the intermediate limbic brain. Emotions can affect how we perceive all these sensations in our conscious brain.

We'll explore this later on when we discuss the structure of our sensory system. For now, here are two major ways the intermediate limbic brain improves our perceptions.

## Improvement of Body Awareness through Internal Body Sensations

This function allows us to feel the status of our intermediate limbic brain. Our intermediate limbic brain perceives sensations from the viscera, our abdominal organs. We call this visceral sensation our "gut feelings." We have no conscious motor control over this system or its sensory perception. Though we might wish we could, we can't make our stomach growl or stop growling at will. The intermediate limbic system does it for us. We do have a subtle conscious perception of these sensations. We feel fear by sensing something in our stomach. Some people, when anxious, can feel a funny sensation in the stomach area or have loose stools or abdominal pain from stimulation of the intermediate limbic motor control on the gut. Two parts of the brain are working together—the new brain's perception of fear as it processes the signals up from the intermediate limbic brain.

## Improvement of Body Awareness and Control through improved Motor Control

The intermediate limbic brain refines our movements and makes them automated, smooth, and unconscious. Again, we won't go into this more here, since this ability has little to do with our topic, love. Here, I mention movements just to illustrate the intermediate limbic brain's effects on us.

What's important to take away is that we have no conscious control over the intermediate limbic brain system or any of its subsystems. More important, without the intermediate limbic brain, we'd live a life as emotionless as that of a lizard sitting on a sunny stump. That lizard doesn't know what fun is, lacking an intermediate limbic brain, but we do.

• • •

Now, since we've finished learning about the old reptilian brain and the intermediate limbic brain, as promised earlier, we'll head over to the third part of the brain—the newest brain, the one that makes us different and exponentially more high-functioning than any other species on the planet.

## New Brain: The Thinking Brain

*(Illustrated in blue )*

The Latin name for the new brain is *neocortex* (*neo* = new, *cortex* = brain cells), hence the term "new neocortex brain" is sometimes used. I will simply refer to this part of the brain as the "new brain."

This, the newest part of the brain, sits above and around the intermediate limbic brain. Looking at it, it seems like it's quite a convoluted arrangement, but developmentally speaking, it's a marvel of efficiency. The new brain kept getting bigger as mammals became more intelligent and eventually became quite big in humans. If measured by comparison to the total body size, the entire brain is ten times bigger in humans

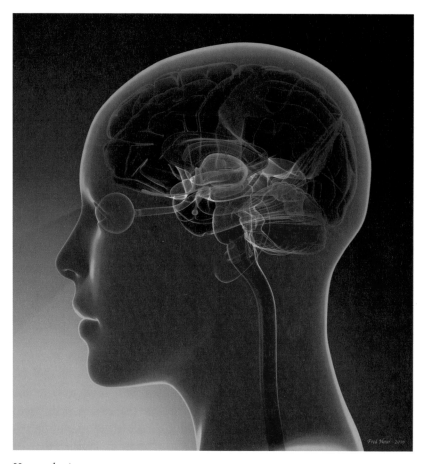

*Human brain*

compared to the old reptilian brain. The new brain is 85 percent of the entire brain. The intermediate limbic brain and the old reptilian brain combined are only 15 percent of the entire brain. The compacted design allows maximum space storage in the limited space of the skull, preventing humans from needing skulls perhaps the size of basketballs to contain all our brain matter.

This new brain allowed for newer abilities; humans acquired new skills such as speaking, understanding spoken words, writing, reading—generally, all forms of language. Mathematics, analysis of information, inventing, and so on are other new skills acquired with the introduction of this new brain. All the wonderful inventions and technological advances are products of this muddled-looking mass.

With the new brain, we acquired much finer motor control with more precise hand dexterity. With the new brain, we acquired exceptionally refined sensory perception of our environment. The new brain is the seat of conscious decisions and conscious perceptions and actions. If there is damage to a person's new brain but the other two parts of the brain are left intact, the person can still protect, rear, and care for his or her children in the usual fashion. Circadian rhythm-related functions are all preserved. The absence of logic, arguments, and volition has no effect on the person's emotional behavior. Only the skills gained by the new brain will be lost, such as language, mathematics, finer motor skills, and so forth.

The new brain has an effect on the intermediate limbic brain, but this effect is weak, and slow. If someone suffers from damage to the intermediate limbic brain, damage that spares the new brain (and of course saves the old reptilian brain so the person can survive), the person's limbic emotions and behaviors are lost. The logic function, the power of argument, and so on will have no value in restoring emotions or emotion-based behavior. That person's relationships with their offspring become just like those seen in reptiles: breed them and forget about them.

Please remember that the old reptilian brain in the crocodile is the same as that in birds and in humans too. Whether human or animal, all have the same old reptilian brain.

The intermediate limbic brains, is almost identical in birds and humans.

If you've ever said, "We aren't animals, we're humans!" that's because humans have the most elaborate, new brain. Our old reptilian brain and intermediate limbic brain are pretty much the same as the one lower animals possess. It's our new brain that makes us different from all other animals.

We've been speaking of only the brain. Now let's look at another vital organ; what you'll learn about it might well surprise you.

## SUMMARY

The oldest brain part is the brain of reptiles, hence called the old reptilian brain. The old reptilian brain keeps our basic organ functions operating: the heart, the lungs, and the digestive system. It's our survival brain.

The next-oldest part of the brain, the intermediate limbic brain, evolved with birds, and gave us quite a few more aspects than simply sur-viving. The intermediate limbic brain added emotions to our brain func-tions and improved our reproduction by introducing the sense of smell to help us identify mates and family. It also introduced emotional interest in our offspring and new emotions for the mate-selection process. It added fear to improve our response to threats. It added an autonomic system to control our bodily functions in relation to needs and introduced joy to our play, eating, socializing, and sex. It started to give us many addictions and compulsions. It introduced a better memory, especially for emotional events, and improved our adaptation to the changing environment by in-troducing the circadian rhythm. This aspect controls hormone release, sleep and fatigue cycles, and our feeding (hunger and satiety) cycle and stabilizes our internal body temperature and internal fluids. The interme-diate limbic brain added emotional effects to our sensations.

The latest part of the brain, the new brain, evolved with late verte-brates and humans. This new brain is our thinking brain, and it's now the largest part of our brains. The new brain introduced language, logic, and analysis and is the seat of conscious decisions and perceptions.

Moving from newest to oldest:

We have one brain part for voluntary intellectual functions, located mainly in the hemispheres of the brain. This is the new brain.

We have another brain part for emotions, located in the intermediate limbic brain. The actions of the intermediate limbic brain are involuntary, with little to no conscious control.

We have a brain part located in the old reptilian brain that keeps us alive but has no emotions or conscious control.

## CHAPTER 4

# LOVE, SEX AND THE HEART

## Love, a Matter of the Heart? Think Again!

Even with our superior intellect and reasoning skills, humans aren't always quick to accept a new theory. In 450 BC Hippocrates proposed, "Emotions emanate from the brain."

It took us a while, but two and a half millennia later, we now know that emotions emanate from the brain.

If we're in love and see our beloved, a lot goes on in the background. We feel excited because the brain releases chemical substances consisting of a group of catecholamines: epinephrine, norepinephrine, dopamine, and also serotonin. This release can make us feel anxious or nervous, or jittery, or have insomnia, and usually, increases sweating. One of these catecholamines, norepinephrine, activates the fight-or-flight response (via the sympathetic nervous system). Catecholamines cause the heart to beat faster and stronger, perceived as palpitations.

While it might seem the heart is the cause of all this flurry of activity, it's not. It's the intermediate limbic brain that sends the signal *down to the heart* to beat faster and harder and for those other manifestations

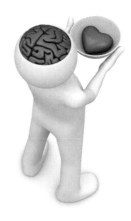

*Is love in the heart or the brain?*

to occur. While it might seem at that moment that the heart is driving the bus, the heart is merely a passive responder to the orders from its master, the brain.

So these symptoms are seen in lovers when they see their beloved. And throughout the ages, until we gained a better understanding of the brain, this was the source of the belief that love comes from the heart. We felt the heart beat faster and stronger, and we (and millions of poets) associated those symptoms with love. But now that science has demystified the real cause of all those fluttering hearts, we know that love comes from the intermediate limbic brain, and the brain chemicals released cause the symptoms in the heart.

Medically, we know that you can't feel or perceive any emotions in the heart. The heart is just a muscle that works as a pump and has a very limited nerve supply and no memory. Some nerves travel down from the brain to the heart. These nerves, as mentioned above, control how fast or slow or how strongly the heart will contract.

Some nerves do go from the heart up to the brain to tell it about what's happening with the heart, but these nerves are mainly pain fibers that, if stimulated, send a pain signal to the brain. You can only feel chest pain, sense the irregular heartbeat, and so on. The heart can't act on its own, so it is only doing what the brain is telling it to do.

Before we leave this small section and head to one at least as interesting to all of us who are interested in love, take a moment to read the love-relevant tidbits we've covered in this chapter so far.

All emotions emanate from the brain. Hippocrates was right. Love comes from the brain but can (and does) manifest itself in the heart.

We shouldn't still be saying, "I love you from the bottom of my heart."

We should be saying, "I love you from the center of my brain" instead!

Even better, say "I love you from the center of my intermediate limbic brain."

That should impress the informed lover!

Now it's time to talk about sex—or at least how the brain contributes to that very large picture.

## Love and the Sex Drive

The sex drive is believed to have existed for five hundred million years. Our sex drive evolved to motivate mate copulation with a range of partners. Genetically speaking, the more partners we mix with, the better offspring we get.

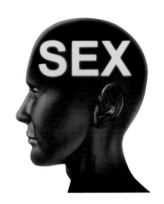

*Sex and the brain*

The sex drive uses separate neuronal (nerve-related) systems from love. It existed much earlier than even the old reptilian brain. As I mentioned before, a documentary about fish reproduction showed a male fish looking right and left continuously to locate fish eggs, and then it dove down to fertilize the eggs and moved on with its search for more eggs to fertilize. Why did Mr. Fish act so off-handedly? Because a fish possesses a sex drive located in its tiny hypothalamus to fertilize eggs, but doesn't know love.

Our intermediate limbic brain, being newer, existed from about one hundred and fifty million years ago, three hundred and fifty million years *after* the sex drive did. When the intermediate limbic brain came along, however, the basic circuitry involved in sex didn't change much. The sex drive was only slightly influenced by the new centers in the intermediate limbic brain and minimally by the new brain.

Sexual desire resides in the hypothalamus. This is the maestro of the intermediate limbic brain, though to look at such a small organ—in adult humans, only the size of an almond—you might not think so. A small portion of this tiny organ is responsible for the sex drive, sexual orientation, and sexual behavior. This portion is called the *medial preoptic area* based on its location in the hypothalamus. It's also called the *sexually dimorphic nucleus* based on its shape. Both names refer to the same hypothalamic part. For simplicity, I'll refer to this part by just one of its names, sexually dimorphic nucleus, or its shortened name, the SDN.

How did such a small spot get such a fancy name? "*Di*" means "two" and "*morphic*" means "shape." It has one shape in males (spherical), and another shape in females (elongated or ovoid). Another common name for the sexually dimorphic nucleus (the SDN) might be of more interest: "the lust center."

Only hormones applied to the sexually dimorphic nucleus will induce sexual behavior, sexual orientation, and sexual desire by releasing dopamine in this miniscule nucleus. Hormonal changes in the body, outside of the brain, have *no* effect on sexual behavior, sexual orientation, or sexual desire.

In all mammals studied, the sexually dimorphic nucleus is at least twice as big in males as in females. This increase in size is caused by the effect *androgens* have on it. Androgens are at least six different hormones; the most famous is one I'm sure you've heard of—testosterone. This increase in size happens when the fetus is eight weeks old. That's the point in gestation when the male testicle starts to make androgens. In that same time period, if androgens don't develop, the fetus becomes a female. Females are programmed differently; the SDN responds to estrogens much later in life, at adolescence, a fact proven in many species in multiple studies.

The difference in size of the sexually dimorphic nucleus between human males and females is much bigger in other animals as well. For you *CSI* fans, yes, we can examine a brain under an electron microscope to determine if this brain belonged to a man or a woman by looking at the size and shape of the SDN. But of course, only after death.

More pertinent to our topic, if this area is damaged, mating behavior is eliminated, as seen in many experiments, and also increasing dopamine in the area causes an increase in sex drive. The sex hormones that induce sex drive and behaviors do so by affecting the sexually dimorphic nucleus. These hormones are mainly androgens. Estrogens are involved too, but the main driver in women is still androgens. Yes, women have androgens in their bodies just like men do, which come from the adrenal gland, the ovaries, fat cells. Androgens are converted to estrogens, and both androgens and estrogens increase during ovulation.

Studies performed on lizards and humans proved that the higher the blood levels of androgens, the higher the sex drive in both sexes, with more frequent sexual activity. We treat patients with low sex drive by giving them androgens. (Note: you might be wondering if the lizard's cold-blooded nature would affect the study results, but it doesn't. There is no difference between cold-blooded species and warm-blooded species in the effect of sex hormones on the sexually dimorphic nucleus.)

Sex hormones also affect our perceptions of the opposite sex by acting on the hypothalamus. Women perceive a man as more attractive when they're ovulating than when they see the same man while menstruating.

The sexually dimorphic nucleus is also involved in sex partner preference. It's known that some male sheep are homosexual. In a homosexual ram, the SDN is half the size of those in heterosexual rams. The *aromatase enzyme*, an enzyme used in the SDN, was found to be twice as high in heterosexual as homosexual rams. Surgically damaging the sexually dimorphic nucleus in heterosexual male ferrets converted them to homosexual ferrets.

Nevertheless, human studies showed conflicting findings. We still don't know for sure what causes homosexuality in humans.

Sexual desire is very powerful and can be destructive to the sex-driven person. Think of the public figures: presidents, presidential candidates, senators, state governors, or celebrated US generals who sullied their reputations because they couldn't control their sexual desires. The downward control from the new brain to the intermediate limbic brain's sexually dimorphic nucleus is sometimes too weak to succeed in inhibiting sexual desire. Their problem was the lack of downward control from the conscious new brain over the lower limbic-brain lust center. In cases like these, the SDN-driven urge for sex overpowers the new brain's logic and values.

The joy of sex is caused by release of monoamines in the sexually dimorphic nucleus, just like in falling in love (romance). Food appetite and sex appetite share the same or similar centers in the hypothalamus, the satiety center.

I recall an incident that happened to me. I was called for a consultation at a psychiatric hospital. The patient was a thirty-five-year-old female with severe, unrelenting headaches. When I went to the nurse's station to find her, I was told, "She's in a group session for sexual obsession, but it will be finished in about five minutes."

Five minutes would give me time to review her chart before meeting her, so that was fine for me. I nodded at the receptionist and took a chair near the meeting room door, where I'd see the group as they left.

In my mind, I was expecting to see a bunch of petite, sexy-looking females with tight clothes and heavy makeup. *Probably most will have lip implants and breast augmentations*, I remember thinking. When the group came out, I was shocked. They were mostly overweight women dressed in ordinary clothes, the type of women you might see every day. I was actually angry about that. I felt that this hospital and the so-called sexual obsession group was a fraud.

Still indignant, I called the psychiatrist who had called for my consultation, to object. "Oh, no," he said, "that's very typical of this disease." He sent me articles that concluded that sufferers of sexual obsession have an overactive "appetite center" or an underactive satiety center in the hypothalamus.

This knowledge was certainly an eye-opening lesson for me. You've no doubt experienced the following: After you eat a big meal, if someone offers you more food, you simply feel you can't eat any more. This is because your satiety center has kicked in to stop you from eating more. The women I saw that day had a weak satiety center that couldn't stop the desire for food, and in the same way, the desire for sex. This desire has nothing to do with true hunger or with love, attachment, or identification. Any food, any mate, is fine. There is no mate selection, no bonding with the mate.

This connection occurs in animals as well. If a male rat smells an estrus (in-heat) female rat, the amount of sex hormones is dramatically increased to stimulate the brain's sex drive and, subsequently, the sex acts. Interestingly, animal studies proved that when the male rat smells the scent of his own female offspring, the sex hormone levels suddenly and dramatically drop. Nature, it seems, has its system for preventing incest. The more involved the male with the care of the offspring, the more the drop of sex hormones.

So, what's love got to do with "it"—with sexual desire? Sexual desire *is* separate from love, though with some overlap.

A correlation here: Doctors have nurses working for them. The doctor has an influence on the nurse. He or she teaches the nurse and guides the nurse in her/his work. The nurse also has influence on the doctor. The nurse helps the doctor to be more efficient by doing many tasks on behalf of the doctor. There is a continuous interaction between them. Yet the doctor is not the nurse and the nurse is not the doctor. It's the same with sex and love.

The sex drive is often expressed toward a range of individuals, while love is expressed toward one specific individual only. (Note: I'm speaking of love in relation to a mate. Love for a mate works within a different brain system from love for parent, children, pets, and so on. All are types of love, but different from the topic here.)

The sex drive is often temporarily suppressed after the sex act (because of the satiety center), whereas lovers never experience that their love is temporarily suppressed after sex. There is no satiety center for love. Everyone wants more love all the time for their entire life.

Many adults get involved in sex with individuals they don't love. The famous individuals mentioned, the politicians and celebrities, most of the time didn't love their sex partners; they just responded to a strong sexual desire. Also, nobody has ever reported that they loved their partner more after receiving androgen boosts for their sex drive!

Some individuals fall madly in love with mates with whom they never had sex. The supposedly true story of "Anna and the King" beautifully illustrates a great sexless love story. Anna and the king never kissed, hugged, or had sex, even though they were madly in love with each other. There is a song in the movie, in fact, that illustrates love without sex.

*Cannot touch, cannot hold, cannot be together*
*Cannot love, cannot kiss, cannot have each other*
*Must be strong and we must let go*
*Cannot say what our hearts must know*

*How can I not love you?*
*What do I tell my heart?*
*When do I not want you,*
*Here in my arms*
*How does one waltz away?*
*From all of the memories*
*How do I not miss you?*
*When you're gone*

*Cannot dream, cannot share, sweet and tender moments*
*Cannot feel, how we feel, must pretend it's over*
*Must be brave and we must go on*
*Must not say what we've known all along.*

If one's sexual advances are rejected, almost no one gets depressed, commits suicide, or kills that rejecting party. In contrast, rejected love causes depressions, suicides, stalking, or even homicide. Love is a much stronger emotion, and could be more destructive than sexual desire.

But again, there is an overlap. The "love chemicals" (monoamines and nonapeptides) stimulate the sex drive indirectly by stimulating the release of sex hormones. Increased sex hormones levels cause increased dopamine release in the sexually dimorphic nucleus, causing more "joy" from sex with the beloved. Orgasm is caused by dopamine release. Orgasm causes the release of nonapeptides and serotonin. Nonapeptides increase the bonding of the couple. Serotonin causes the post-sex calming effect and stimulates the satiety center, thus suppressing further desire for sex but not for love.

Some call the sex drive *lust* or *intimacy*. Some writers believe that this is the first phase of love. I disagree.

## SUMMARY

Sex evolved three hundred and fifty million years before love. The sex drive comes from our hypothalamus, a part of the intermediate limbic brain stimulated by sex hormones. That location in the hypothalamus is called the sexually dimorphic nucleus, the SDN. The effects of androgens (hormones) on the SDN cause the sex drive, sexual orientation, and sexual behavior. Love can stimulate the sex drive by releasing more hormones, sex enhances love by releasing monoamines and nonapeptides.

The sex drive is suppressed by the satiety center. The satiety center does not suppress love. Love makes sex feel a lot better and more satisfying, but love is not sex, and sex is not love. You can have sex with someone you don't love. You can also love someone without ever having sex with them.

*Love does not start with lust.*
*Love is not lust and lust is not love.*

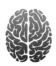

## CHAPTER 5

# PHASE ONE OF LOVE—FINDING THE PERSON OF MY DREAMS

When I was a neurology resident at the Baylor College of Medicine, we had a daily six p.m. lecture about topics in neurology. These lectures were held in a large conference room with a big long table in the middle, where we residents sat. A faculty member would arrive and stand by the end of the table, a projector screen behind him, and teach us about the details of a specific topic.

One afternoon, a faculty neurosurgeon was coming to teach us about the techniques and technologies they use to avoid injury to important brain structures during brain operations. He had a nurse call us and tell us that his last case was taking longer than expected, but he would finish the surgery and then come over to give us the lecture. We split into a few groups around the table, each discussing different topics.

Near my end of the table, a resident named Debbie talked to another resident, John, and I couldn't help overhearing.

"Have you met the new psych resident?" Debbie said. "He's the man of my dreams. Six feet tall, a slim figure, and gorgeous blond hair and blue eyes."

Chuckling, John replied, "Do you always specify the body dimensions for the man of your dreams?"

Debbie nodded, sharing the laugh. "Yes, and in fine detail."

It was time for me to jump in. "I can't believe you have such a well-defined physical image of your dream lover," I said. "Me, I just define her as having acceptable looks, pretty if possible, but my main feature of attraction is intelligence."

Debbie shrugged. "Of course I want him to be intelligent. But if he doesn't have the physical characteristics I want, no matter how intelligent, he's disqualified."

Before I had the chance to tease her about being so forthright, another resident, an attractive and brilliant woman named Nicole, chimed in. "I know what you mean, Debbie. In South America where I'm from, we like macho men. I dream of a man with big, strong muscles, who'll physically fight for me and protect me if I need him to. And sure, intelligence matters, but if he isn't macho, forget it!"

I groaned. "You two have to be kidding. The days of physical labor and needing physical protection are gone. I thought nowadays women want the intellect, not the physique. Brains not brawn, get it?"

Nicole rolled her eyes at me, though in a friendly way. "Both are important," she said, "but still … what a guy looks like is really important to me."

A resident named Susan had been studying her notes—we residents were almost always studying—but at this, she dropped her pen onto her folder and huffed impatiently. "I cannot believe that you *intelligent* people care about physical looks. My dream man is all defined based on his personality. I don't care if he's tall or short, fat or skinny, has big muscles or no muscles at all. What good is all that if I'm bored with him? I want to be intellectually stimulated all the time. That's my dream man."

Nicole sighed. "Well, I know that all men want a woman with big breasts and an hourglass figure. Nothing else matters to men. They just want a sex object."

John must have decided it was time to take back control. "Look, sex is important, so I want a woman who can offer that. But if she's dumb, I'll be turned off. I broke up with a few girls because they weren't able to engage in a stimulating conversation. The sex was a good attraction, at first, but that wore out quickly. I just couldn't stay with a woman who could only offer sex."

Nicole grinned his way. "You must be a *very* rare exception, then."

John turned to me. "Hey, you're a guy. Do you agree with me?"

I was spared from having to answer when the neurosurgery professor walked into the room. But the question and what came before it stayed with me to this day.

So:

- Do you have a picture of the person of your dreams in your mind?
- Is the image defined by specific, detailed physical characteristics? By intellectual characteristics? A combination of both?
- When did you start forming this image of the person of your dreams? Was it last week, or maybe just in the last few years? Or did you start building the image much earlier?
- What determines the details of this mental image? Is it your genes? Your upbringing? Is it your previous experiences with other people? All of the above?
- When, how, and why do we begin to form this mental image?

The answers to all or most of the questions can be found in our brains. Do you know this song by the group Foreigner?

*Waiting for a girl like you for so long*
*I've been looking too hard, I've been waiting too long*
*Sometimes I don't know what I will find*
*I only know it's a matter of time*
*When you love someone*
*It feels so right, so warm and true*
*I need to know if you feel it too*
*Maybe I'm wrong*
*Won't you tell me if I'm coming on too strong?*
*This heart of mine has been hurt before*
*This time I wanna be sure*
*I've been waiting for a girl like you*
*To come into my life*
*I've been waiting for a girl like you*
*A love that will survive*
*I've been waiting for someone new*
*To make me feel alive*
*You're so good*
*When we make love it's understood*
*It's more than a touch or a word we say*

*Only in dreams could it be this way*
*When you love someone*
*Yeah, really love someone*
*Now, I know it's right*
*From the moment I wake up till deep in the night*
*There's nowhere on earth that I'd rather be*
*Than holding you, tenderly*
*I've been waiting for a girl like you to come into my life*
*I've been waiting for a girl like you*
*And a love that will survive*
*I've been waiting for someone new*
*To make me feel alive*
*Yeah, waiting for a girl like you*
*To come into my life*
*I've been waiting, waiting for you, ooh*
*Ooh, I've been waiting*
*I've been waiting, yeah*
*I've been waiting for a girl like you*
*I've been waiting*
*Won't you come into my life?*
*My life?*
*For you are mine*
*At last.*

Do you remember when you started dreaming about that special someone?

When one of my daughters was six years old, we attended a wedding. In the pew beside me, she sat in the gorgeous church, gazing around, admiring its beauty. Without warning, she looked at me and said, "Dad, please help me remember where this church is."

I understood part of her question: that church wasn't in our neighborhood. What I didn't understand was the *why* of her request. When I asked her, she said, "Because this church is so beautiful, I'm going to get married in it!"

Hiding my mirth at her statement, I said, "So … do you know whom you're going to marry?"

"Of course not," she said. "I'm only six years old. But I know when I grow up I'll marry someone. I want to get married in this beautiful church!"

Two years later, during another wedding, she chose the wedding reception hall as where she would have her wedding reception when she married.

My other daughter didn't choose a church or a wedding reception locale. At age five, after attending a wedding where the groom was dressed in a bowtie, she chose a man to marry, and announced her choice to me

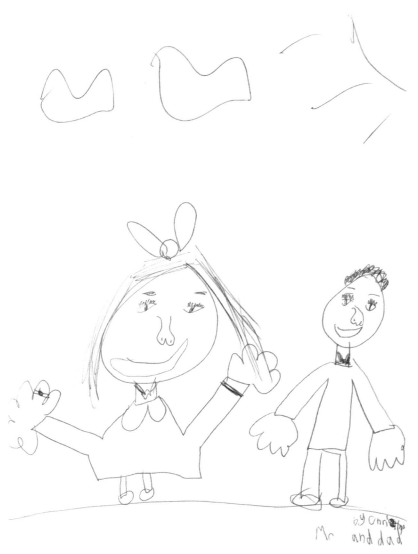

*My daughter's wedding plan*

with a picture. She'd drawn an image of herself wearing a white dress and a necklace, and with a ring on her left ring finger. Next to her, wearing a bowtie, was the man of her dreams. The best man she ever met. That man was me.

## The Mate Selection Process

We start to prepare for falling in love, romantic love, at a very young age, perhaps as soon as we're able to have awareness of our environment, and far in advance of the need to select a mate for reproduction. How did this mate selection process we have today come about?

### Benefits of Sexual Reproduction

Sexual reproduction happens when the sperm's DNA (male genes) and the egg's DNA (female genes) mix to form a *zygote* (a single-cell fetus that will grow into a full fetus in about nine months). This mixing of DNA genes from the sperm and the egg causes two sets of DNA genes, one set from each parent, to combine into one set of genes in the offspring, the fetus.

We call this the *recombination* of two sets of genes into a single set of mixed genes.

Recombination offers many advantages to the offspring, especially in improving and repairing genetic defects. We can repair gene defects by *copying* good genes over bad genes, or *hiding* the bad genes and using only the good genes. We can *combine* two talents, one from the mother and one from the father, to have a child with "double talent." The children of that new child will all continue to have the double talents.

*The goal of love is reproduction, producing healthier or improved offspring.*

Mate selection is unconsciously controlled by the desire to get good genes from the chosen mate. You'll learn how this unconscious selection happens later on, when we discuss the effect of genes (DNA) on mate selection.

## Further Advances in Mate Selection

The mate-selection process continued to improve with further development of the brain. New genes developed that help us to select a preferred mate, for better genetic pool selection.

This mate selection process involves three phases of selection.

The resident doctors in the story I told you a bit ago were trying to describe how they would choose their best mate, the person of their dreams. This imagining is *pre-coital (sex) selection*, the first phase.

Men are done with selection process once they select the best woman they can find and give her their genes.

Women don't stop there, though; biologically speaking, they continue to select the best sperm out of fifty million, the ballpark number of sperm in a single ejaculation. All fifty million will race from the cervix to the fallopian tubes. Only the fastest will arrive there first. This is selecting during the sex act, known as *intracoital selection*.

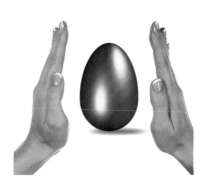

So are women done selecting at that point? No, they aren't. The woman's body unconsciously monitors the development of the fetus, and if it's not good enough, the body will spontaneously miscarry the fetus early in the pregnancy, so she will get pregnant again soon with a better fetus. We still don't know how

*Woman holding her golden egg*

the female body detects the genes in the fetus but know that they do so, and reliably. So women are still selecting, even after getting pregnant. This is *postcoital* selection.

*Women are very fussy about their valuable golden egg.*

Before coitus, women and men select the mate with the best genes.

During coitus, women select the best genes their chosen mate can offer.

After coitus, women's bodies check the outcome of the selection. If she has bad genes, she miscarries that bad fetus.

*The purpose of love is to produce the healthiest offspring ever conceived.*

Now, let's look at the details of this; let's understand how the selection process continued to become more sophisticated with the more elaborate brain parts by looking at precoital selection of various classes of animals.

- Precoital selection in animals with an old reptilian brain
- Precoital selection in animals with an intermediate limbic brain
- Precoital selection in animals with the new brain

*Understanding mate selection evolution will help us understand how we choose a mate now.*

## Precoital Mate Selection in Reptiles (Old Reptilian Brain)

In frogs, studies found that the female frog selects males with wider bodies and deeper cloacae (mating pouches), over the opposites. Wider bodies mean better genes for body development. Deep cloacae mean more sperm stored, assuring better fertility chances. Unlike that group of earth's residents, there is no dreaming and no preplanning for meeting a mate, just picking the best available mate at the opportune time. The females base their choices on visual selection. In an experiment, scientists changed the visual effects on the selection scene. They found that if they changed the white light at the mating scene to a blue light, the female choices changed.

Female frogs visually scan males for better genes (healthier offspring) and higher copulation chances (more offspring with better genes). They use sound in a similar way, to screen for stronger voices (better genes). In the study, females preferred males with stronger voices.

If you look at today's dating websites, you find that mates still look at the chosen sex's pictures before wanting to know anything else about them. Many potential mates are instantaneously rejected based on this visual scanning method. Most mates still unconsciously look for the same criteria in a match, for the mate who appears to have good genes (handsome/beautiful) and looks sexier (higher fertility chances). This behavior is seen even if the display-choosers (person looking for a mate) are post-reproduction age. Almost all post-menopausal women, who cannot have children, still look for a handsome and potentially fertile (sexy) man.

We humans have nearly the same old reptilian brain structures. We still choose a mate in the same way reptiles do.

## Precoital Selection in Birds (Intermediate Limbic Brain)

With the development of the intermediate limbic brain, things got more sophisticated.

Male sperm stayed smaller and larger in numbers. Female eggs became bigger, so they became fewer in number. Females had fewer chances to get the better genes for better offspring with these changes, so females had to develop a more sophisticated process for selecting the best male partner for their valuable egg.

We've learned about how reptiles choose their mates. How do birds choose the best mate?

Various systems have developed in animals over time. In all the systems, there are two parties. The exhibitor, usually the male, shows off his good genes and high fertility potential in various ways. The selector, usually the female, screens all the offers before choosing the best mate for the job.

*Using emotions to select a mate is the beginning of the feelings of love.*

A common example is the *peacock*. Peacocks are one part of a bird family called *peafowls*. In this family the male is called a peacock, the female is called a *peahen*, and the offspring are *peachicks*. At mating time, peacocks, the males, will walk around the females exhibiting their large, colorful tail feathers. Females, the peahens, will visually select for mating the males with the best, largest, most colorful display. This selection phase is done by screening multiple potential partners for the best mate and uses many of the peahen's senses as well as stored memories in the peahen's intermediate limbic brain.

Eyespots are the colored circles in the peacock's tail, and the number of these varies among various peacocks. Females are proven to select the males with the largest number of eyespots. In studies, removing eyespots from some peacocks caused them to be less favored by females. Do

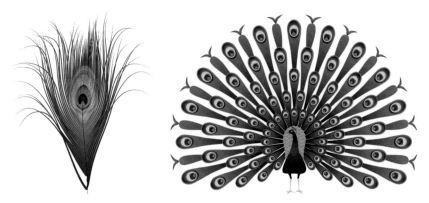

*Peacock eyespots*        *Peacock*

peahens know what they're doing? Yes. Peachicks fathered by the more ornamented males weighed more than those fathered by less ornamented males, an attribute generally associated with a better survival rate in birds. Peachicks fathered by more ornamented males, when grown up, also survived predators better than peachicks fathered by the less ornamented males. Peahens knew what they were doing!

> *Females have such good eyes for good mates, their mate selections proved a very reliable method for detecting better genes in male partners.*

This example demonstrates how bird mating differs from that of reptiles. Female peahens use sensory perceptions (vision, hearing and smell), memory of other peacocks (where selection criteria were stored in the intermediate limbic brain), and emotions too. Emotions in the intermediate limbic brain cause the peahen to be motivated to pursue the courtship of the chosen peacock (in the mating dance). She selects, then flirts and courts him into action—or perhaps we should we say she *seduces* him into action. Frogs don't flirt, court, or seduce.

## Precoital Selection in Humans (New Brain)

Now we can discuss that group of resident doctors' mate selection ideas.

In primitive species, the courtship attractions last for minutes, hours, days, or at most, weeks. In humans, however, it takes many years to reproduce a healthy, independent offspring. So, in humans, mate selection evolved further by incorporating the new brain in the mate selection process.

The first phase is simply about choosing a mate. Now, with the conscious new brain, we can also involve our intellect in the mate selection process.

Mate selection in humans starts with screening, and the selection ends by falling in love. That moment of falling in love ends phase one of love and starts phase two.

*Falling in love represents the finalization of mate selection.*

Why do humans have to prepare in advance for mate selection? When humans choose a mate, they use two brain parts: a new brain, which is conscious, and an innate, unconscious intermediate limbic brain.

The new brain selects features related to the chosen mate's new brain, such as similar intelligence, common interests, and common family backgrounds. The personality of the mate is important, "personality" being defined as the potential mate's style of behavior. We want someone with compatible personality so we can get along. From a young age, humans start to form a mental image—termed *fantasia*[4] in Latin—of "the Person of My Dreams," in intermediate limbic brain memory. This mental image/fantasia is partly instinctual, determined by genes inherited from reptiles and birds, and partially conscious, determined by our conscious new brain.

We continually refine the stored fantasia (intermediate limbic brain data or memory) of the perfect potential mate. As we meet more people with features we desire to have in our future mates, the stored image of our Person of My Dreams, our fantasia, is refined further still.

Do you remember when you started liking members of the other sex and thinking, *This one is cute, I want to marry someone like him/her*? Of course this wasn't the end of the search but the nascent beginning.

In earlier societies let's use the Middle Ages as an example we met few potential mates that we wanted to incorporate in our fantasia. A typical village person might meet four to six new people in a lifetime that they'd

---

4. The word *fantasia* evolved in the English cultures to mean dreaming or imagining. In Latin it was used to mean a mental image of reality.

like to incorporate in their fantasia. Finding a mate with these features was relatively easy then, with so few choices. My young daughter found a mate easily at age five, the best man she'd met so far in her life, her wonderful dad. Now that she's older, I doubt I'm still her fantasia.

Since I'm neither a psychiatrist nor a psychologist, I won't delve into the psychology behind "how to choose the perfect mate" further. There are many excellent books that deal with this component and have been written by specialists in that field. I will only give you, later on, my own perception on this.

We've been talking about the new brain system of mate selection. Now let's move to the next system.

As you've learned, the second system is the intermediate limbic brain. The instinctual part uses inherited and saved gene programs in our intermediate limbic brain that guide us to select the best precoital mate based on their good genes and reproductive potential. This uses the same system used by reptiles and birds. We call mates with high reproductive potential "sexy." Both sexes want a mate who is healthy and sexy. This is done unconsciously by being attracted to certain mates. There is a strong effect from our genes on this selection, and I'll discuss the role played by our genes later on.

The new brain has a downward connection to the intermediate limbic brain, but this connection is weak, and slow. It's possible to cross over a poorly constructed or very old rope bridge, but as any hiker knows, it's best to take the crossing with great care. Doing so increases the chance of making it to the other side without incident. To influence the intermediate limbic brain in mate selection, we use this weak downward connection slowly, over many years and over many life experiences. To accomplish this by our peak reproductive years, we start early in life.

Next, you'll see how we unconsciously select that mate who will help us produce the healthiest offspring, with a further look into how humans make the mate selection using the above instinct and their conscious brain.

### Attraction in Humans: Precoital Selection of an Attractive Mate

Let's consider some studies done about mate selection in humans.

In one study about our selection of "attractive mates," each sex was shown pictures of the opposite sex and asked to rate their attractiveness and give them a score between 1 and 10, where 10 is the perfect mate.

Western ideas, the Indian divorce rate has dramatically increased to one in one hundred. Still, this is better than the Western model, with its divorce rate of forty to fifty per one hundred marriages.

The numbers are clear; there is a much lower divorce rate among arranged marriages. How is it possible that two mates preselected to marry each other are more successful?

I had to ask doctors who were in arranged marriages to try to understand the reason.

When asking them about the details of their fantasia, I found interesting differences. Hinduism has set up a system for family and marriage. Hindu doctrine prohibits young men and women from participating in mate selection, and restricts that process to the parents. There's also a caste system, and everyone is expected to marry someone from his or her own caste. This caste system seems to minimize the difference in values and culture between future mates.

They also have a dowry system where the bride's family pays for the groom. Hearing this, I recalled asking a female Indian doctor about her fantasia image. I asked if she ever dreamed of marrying a man who looked and talked like her country's best movie stars. I was surprised when she laughed and said, "My parents could never afford the dowry of such a perfect man. I knew what my parents could afford, and dreamed within their limits. It's like when you're going to college and need a car. You see all the beautiful Ferraris, but you know your parents can only afford a used Honda. You dream about your used Honda, not the Ferrari."

Another doctor told me that his wife was chosen for him when he was a child. He said he grew up dreaming about sharing love with her, and tried many times to sneak over the wall around her house to see her playing with friends and often thought how happy he would be when he married her. He and his wife grew up setting their fantasia to be that of an already-identified person. All the dreams of happiness were well defined in their minds, and they knew happiness would come when they were with this identified person. No need to idealize a movie star or TV host. In effect, "I already know who is my prince or princess."

There is also no remarrying, ever. If the mate dies, the widow cannot remarry. Every person has only one mate for their lifetime. It's not surprising, then, that they feel they should take good care of that mate, or they'll be alone for the rest of their lives.

Every one of these people I talked with told me they fell in love, fell out of love, and grew into True Love, just like the Western model. Their only difference was their fantasia.

In my view, the reason for the higher success rate of relations in the arranged-marriage countries is the way they set up the first phase of love, the programming for selecting the Person of My Dreams, the fantasia. They program their young ones to accept what they get rather than dream about the perfect mate. While no longer possible in the United States, if there ever was a way, I wish we could see how our children would select a mate with a reality-based fantasia.[5]

• • •

So we're finished with the precoital selection of a mate in reptiles, birds, and humans, and the fussy human female and male have chosen the best genes they could find.

Is it over yet? It is for males, at least from a scientific standpoint, but not for females.

During intracoital selection, the man and woman fell in love and are ready to consummate the relationship. Are females done selecting now? No. As mentioned before, the female body is perfectly designed to make it difficult for all but the strongest, and therefore healthiest, sperm to reach and impregnate that valuable egg.

In postcoital selection, the egg is now fertilized, and the female is pregnant. Is she done with mate selection? No, she's not. As earlier described and by a process we don't yet know, the female body somehow monitors the growth of that fertilized egg. If the fetus turns out to have bad genes, her body rejects it through a spontaneous miscarriage, and so the process of selection begins anew.

Perhaps now, recalling the story of Inanna and Dumuzi (the poem from earlier), it seems more understandable that Inanna, the girl in the poem, would be so choosy when deciding between the two potential mates—the biological drive to settle for nothing less than the best possible match has been around as long as the human brain! In fact, it seems a good time to return to Inanna and Dumuzi's story to answer the question, has love changed in the last four thousand years?

You recall how Inanna initially rejected the unknown shepherd for

---

5. There has been no research on that topic, as far as I know. I wish we could study this further.

the familiar farmer. The farmer was local, but the shepherd was from another kingdom.

*Nay, the man of my heart is he*
*Who has won my heart is he*
*The one who hoes,*
*His grain storehouses are heaped high,*
*The grain is brought regularly into the storehouse,*
*The farmer, he whose grain that fills all the grain storehouse*

*I—the shepherd I will not marry,*
*I will not wear his coarse garments, I will not accept his coarse wool,*

*I, the maid, the farmer I will marry,*
*The farmer who grows many plants,*
*The farmer who grows much grain.*

Oh, my. Should Inanna marry the farmer with his heaps of grain, or the shepherd with his coarse wool?

"Who is my ideal mate?" she is saying. "The farmer? The shepherd? I have to choose just one but which one?"

While the mate-selection drive was surely at work as well, I believe that she didn't love the farmer. She just thought that he was more familiar to her and thus a safer option. When we discuss "falling in love" in more depth, I'll prove to you that she fell in love with the shepherd. If she loved the farmer, she would have felt that the shepherd was repulsive.

When she preferred the farmer, she hadn't yet met the shepherd in person. Inanna made mate selection sight unseen. Luckily for her, she had only two options. Modern lovers have many more mates to choose from, which makes the choice much harder. As happens in other areas of life, sometimes many choices make it impossible to select just one.

Whether the choice is among many or only two, we all decide very quickly about a potential mate's suitability for us. We call it *chemistry*, and as you'll see in a bit, this isn't an incorrect way to describe it. In scant seconds and with visual, auditory, and olfactory (smell) scanning, we decide, "Yes I am interested," or "No thanks, that isn't what I'm looking for." We make a very quick but definitive decision. Only after Dumuzi convinced Inanna's new brain that he was as good as the farmer, and that his pedigree was as esteemed as hers, did she accept him as a viable option for her and agree to go out on a date with him—what passed for a date in ancient times, you might say. She made a mate selection.

*When Inanna finalized her mate selection,*
*she fell in love with Dumuzi.*

## SUMMARY

Mate selection is all about better gene selection. Selection involves three stages of selection: precoital, intracoital, and postcoital. To improve the precoital selection process further, we developed an attraction system. Old reptilian brains used visual and auditory methods. With the intermediate limbic brain, love and its emotions emerged. We developed a monoamines-based system of selection (attraction) to finalize the mate selection and cause us to feel that we fell in love. We also developed a nonapeptides-based system for bonding the pairs for longer periods by inducing True Love. With new brain evolution, our mate selection improved further by incorporating our best experiences into the Person of My Dreams image that is stored in our intermediate limbic brain. We all decide very quickly about our mate's suitability for us by using our intermediate limbic brain, and we call it chemistry. In a few seconds and with visual scanning, mainly, we decide, "Yes I'm interested" or "No thanks, that isn't what I'm looking for." We make a very quick but definitive decision. We then allow the new brain to make further decisions on our preselected mate. With the consent of the intermediate limbic brain and the new brain, we finalize the mate selection and immediately start the next phase of love: we fall in love with that chosen mate.

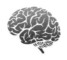

## CHAPTER 6

# PHASE TWO OF LOVE—
# ROMANTIC LOVE CHEMICALS:
# MONOAMINES

---

William Shakespeare once said, "Love is merely a madness."

Is love a madness? The better question might be, why do lovers act so differently when in love than when not in love? Why do they bounce between exhilaration, euphoria, increased energy, sleeplessness, loss of appetite, trembling, a racing heart, and accelerated breathing, as well as anxiety, panic, and despair when the relationship suffers even the smallest setback?

Could all of this be explained by monoamines?

| Love Chemicals Summary | | |
|---|---|---|
| **Family** | **Children** | **Grandchildren** |
| Monoamines | Catecholamines | Epinephrine |
| | | Norepinephrine |
| | | Dopamine |
| | Serotonin | Serotonin |

As we discussed before, monoamines are a family with two children. One is called catecholamines, which has three members: epinephrine, norepinephrine, and dopamine. The other child is called serotonin. The catecholamines play important roles in the process of falling in love, so I'll describe each one now. We will follow this catecholamine discussion by talking about the other child, serotonin.

## Epinephrine

The emotional effects of epinephrine include enhancing the sense of fear and other negative feelings. I'm sure you'll agree these aren't typical features of normal love. Other effects of epinephrine, however, are related to love. Epinephrine enhances the long-term recall of emotionally charged memories. That's how we're able to remember our first kiss. Jealousy, paranoia, shakiness, anxiety, and sweating seen in this phase of love are caused by epinephrine.

## Norepinephrine

Norepinephrine is present in different parts of the body. The part that matters to us is, of course, the brain. Norepinephrine's main "brain center" is located in the middle of the old reptilian brain, in the *locus ceruleus*, which literally means "the blue location." The locus ceruleus was discovered in 1786 because of its noticeable blue color seen on brain slices, but research on it was delayed for a long time due to the extremely small connections it has, which were actually invisible until 1959, when a Swedish scientist found a way to stain the cells and see the connections. Actually, most useful research started after 1969. This time lag resulted in a relative paucity of knowledge about its functions in the brain compared to other neurotransmitters.

Yet, we still know many things about it. The locus ceruleus sends connections to almost all brain centers.

I've said that the hypothalamus is the maestro of the intermediate limbic brain, and now I can say that the locus ceruleus is probably the maestro of the three brain parts, the central command center for the old reptilian brain, intermediate limbic brain, and new brain. We usually refer to it as the *locus ceruleus-norepinephrine*, where "locus ceruleus" is the name of the "house" (the location) and "norepinephrine" (the neurotransmitter) is the name of the "resident" in that same house, somewhat like saying John Smith of 123 Main Street.

The locus ceruleus receives information from many brain centers, but the locus ceruleus has no or very limited connections to the hypothalamus, where our sex drive resides. This could explain why some people have weakness when it comes to consciously suppressing sexual urges, as we will see later.

So, what does this norepinephrine-making locus ceruleus do for love?

When they see their lover, lovers in romance lose sleep, are more attentive to their lover, and feel their heart beating faster and stronger. We can also explain why lovers during romance have dilated eyes, which is the effect the locus ceruleus has on the loving mate. During romance, phase two of love, locus ceruleus-norepinephrine prepares us to have an intense True Love in phase four of love.

The best way to explain how the locus ceruleus works to affect our brain functions is to use an analogy. We'll use our government and its goals.

### Goal: Search for changes in the environment and forward the information to the interested party.

Like America's Central Intelligence Agency, the CIA, the locus ceruleus receives multiple pieces of information sent to it from various sources—although in the case of the CIA, those sources tend to include reports from spies, electronic surveys, satellites, and so forth. The CIA continuously searches for new, useful information that can help the country succeed and be safe. This is the *search* phase, which uses *information-in* data.

The locus ceruleus receives information from all our senses and receives this array of sensory information from the old brain, intermediate limbic brain, and new brain, which it uses to *search* for changes in the environment. This is the locus ceruleus *information-in* connection.

The information gathered by the CIA is sent to the various departments, depending on the data's significance and subject. Some data will go to the Department of Defense, State Department, or whatever place it might be most needed. This sending of data is *information-out*. With the locus ceruleus, *information-out* connects to other parts of the brain.

So, the locus ceruleus searches for new information from all brain parts, then forwards it to the correct brain center that needs the information.

The CIA continuously scans the environment for changes that can affect the country's safety or that give chances for better gains in the current world environment. The CIA's goal is to avoid harm and maximize benefits to the country.

If the CIA identifies a threat to the country, such as news that a foe is making nuclear weapons, the CIA will place the lion's share of its focus on this new threat and ignore other routine information.

When the locus ceruleus detects a change in the environment, it increases attention to the new change and suppresses attention to other factors.

When we're searching for the perfect mate, we're using that locus ceruleus-norepinephrine system to scan for potential mates, then select a target—a mate—and focus all our attention on that potential mate. All other mates are ignored, based on norepinephrine's effect.

### Goal: Pay attention to opportunity and risks.

The CIA wants to make sure no mistakes happen, so it has to keep appropriate departments on alert for new information. If departments aren't alert, the usefulness of their gathered data could be impaired.

The locus ceruleus, via norepinephrine release, does the same. When locus ceruleus activity is up, more norepinephrine is released, so the entire brain is more alert and attentive to changes in the environment and performs better and more accurately during tasks such as steering a car. When the locus ceruleus firing decreases, there is less accuracy in tasks performed and more drowsiness. We call this the locus ceruleus-norepinephrine effect on attention.

So, locus ceruleus-norepinephrine hyperactivity is responsible for the lack of sleep common to lovers in the romantic phase of love, and during that phase, the lovers have dilated pupils; both findings were studied and proven in humans and many animals. The locus ceruleus causes us to be more attentive to our beloved mate.

The locus ceruleus information-out sends signals that go from the locus ceruleus to the autonomic nervous system (these "electrical cables" are called the sympathetic chain). When a lover in phase two of love sees the beloved, the locus ceruleus activity increases, thus releasing more norepinephrine. The sympathetic nerves that go to the heart release norepinephrine and epinephrine there, which is responsible for getting their heart to beat faster and stronger, which makes the lover feel that his/her heart is coming out of his/her chest. Again, love resides in the brain, not the heart.

### Goal: Orchestrate good communication across the entire system to help good decisions be made.

When information carried by *fibers* (tiny electric wires) travels from lower brain levels to higher brain centers, we call this *bottom-up* connection (CIA to the president); when it moves from the president to, say, lower-level cabinet members, this is *top-down* connection.

This new, important information from the CIA has to go to a decision center (the president), or in the case of the locus ceruleus, to the *prefrontal cortex* in the brain. The president (prefrontal cortex) makes decisions—for example, whether to move military forces or start an economic embargo— or in the case of the brain, whether to pursue or ignore a potential mate.

Once the president makes a decision, he will execute it by sending commands down the chain of command, for example to the Secretary of Defense and Secretary of State. These are top-down commands.

Decisions made in the prefrontal cortex ("the president") are sent down to two other new-brain centers, asking them to execute the decisions. These two new brain centers are known as the *orbitofrontal cortex* ("Secretary of Defense") and the *anterior cingulate cortex* ("Secretary of State").

The orbitofrontal cortex is proven to enhance the pursuit of *rewards*: joy, pleasure, and so on. This is the center that tells you, "Go for the fun, don't stop, you only live once, take risks, you are indomitable." This "Secretary of Defense" wants to start a war to seek more advantage over the foe? Not a problem. This is probably the site where drug addiction behavior starts.

The other center, the anterior cingulate cortex ("Secretary of State"), does something different. This part of the brain is proven to *inhibit* the pursuit of rewards, joy, pleasure, and so forth, by recalling all the negative experiences we had in the past; that is *risk aversion*. Remember the war the Secretary of Defense was so eager to start? Not this Secretary of State, who will recall the losses from past wars. This is the center that tells you "Don't go all the way for the fun, stop and think about the harm you learned from the past. This can hurt you, too! You want to play it safe and avoid too much risk." The anterior cingulate cortex also receives information from the intermediate limbic brain centers and is the link between the new brain and the intermediate limbic brain. This connection could be how we make mate selection choices. Our instincts want us to be careful, and not take too much risk with our valuable genes or the golden egg.

The final command will be a compromise between taking too much risk (the orbitofrontal cortex, or Secretary of Defense) and taking no risk at all (the anterior cingulate cortex, or Secretary of State). Now we take limited risks and send the command to the locus ceruleus to be executed by all branches of government, or all brain systems. Sorry, but here we have to assume that it's the CIA that organizes the final execution of orders from the president.

### Goal: Influence other systems for your benefit.

The locus ceruleus modulates other brain chemical systems.

The effect of the locus ceruleus on other brain systems is called *modulation*. Oprah modulated her shows, using her skills to make one guest, then another, more active and talk while the other was silent. She modulated by suppressing one side, then activating it, while doing the opposite for the other side. This is modulation.

Locus ceruleus connects the emotion centers in the intermediate limbic brain to the emotion-processing centers in the new brain: the prefrontal cortex, the orbitofrontal cortex, and the anterior cingulate cortex. This is probably how our intermediate limbic brain affects our conscious "love behavior."

Recently, a woman told me that she'd met a man who was attractive and "sexy" but a total mismatch for her intellectually and financially. She divorced a previous husband because he was an alcoholic, but this new man drank even more. Upset with herself, she decided she would terminate the relationship with the new man and never see him again. Only minutes after the decision, he texted her to come over, and she jumped into her car to go to him, unable to stop herself from going. Could this inability have been from the strong signal from the intermediate limbic brain, to the locus ceruleus, to the new brain, forcing the desire to drive to his house against her will? Driving is a new brain function, but something like that could be against our will at times.

The locus ceruleus works by increasing or decreasing (modulating) the activity of *other* neurotransmitters. Norepinephrine is known to enhance both the numbers of nonapeptides making cells and the number of receptors on the nonapeptide-receiving cells, causing an increase in nonapeptides expression. Nonapeptides are responsible for phase four of love, True Love. Thus, earlier release of norepinephrine during phase two of love increases the intensity of the "true love feelings" seen in phase four of love. Romance is a preparatory phase for True Love. This is the reason why those who marry for money, without falling in love, never experience True Love.

Locus ceruleus-norepinephrine has connections with the appetite center, which could explain the loss of appetite for those in phase two of love.

The locus ceruleus-norepinephrine system affects our social-emotional responses—how we emotionally react to certain social events by feeling happy or stressed, depending on the circumstances of the social interaction. This, again, is the compromise of downstream effects from the orbitofrontal cortex and the anterior cingulate cortex.

So, could the formation of our fantasia, the image of our ideal mate, be heavily dependent on this locus ceruleus-norepinephrine connection? Most likely it is, but the research on fantasia is in its infancy still.

We know that the locus ceruleus has connections to the dopamine centers in a two-way communication. Thus, the locus ceruleus affects dopamine, and dopamine can affect the locus ceruleus.

The locus ceruleus also has connections to serotonin centers in the brain. Locus ceruleus-norepinephrine affects serotonin levels. Norepinephrine is actually a target for treating serotonin-deficiency disorders, such as depression. (We'll discuss this later when we discuss serotonin's role in love.)

**Goal: Continue monitoring for new opportunities and risk.**

Once the threat from a foe is over, such as that sudden threat of a nuclear war I mentioned, the CIA will go back to scanning everything for any changes and will react to new changes in the same way as before. In summary, we humans have an *information-in* to the decision center, and an *information-out* system, both of which return to the *search* for new changes by using more *information-in* connections, decisions, and so on. Applied to love, once a potential mate is identified, we focus on the new potential mate, judge their worthiness, and move forward, or go back to search mode. If the potential mate turns out to be a bad choice, we use the locus ceruleus system to ignore him or her and start looking all over again.

We're now finished with the first two members of the catecholamines, epinephrine and norepinephrine. Next, let's learn about the third and last member of the catecholamine family, dopamine.

## Dopamine

If some manifestations of falling in love are caused in part by an excess dopamine effect, then understanding how dopamine works and where it's located in our brain should help us understand how we get many of those wondrous falling-in-love feelings. I use the phrase "dopamine effect" because an increase in dopamine-induced behavior is kind of like knowing whether the car might be going slower because we pushed less hard on the accelerator, because we pushed harder on the brakes, or because we switched to a lower transmission gear. We can't always say with confidence which action caused the slowing, so we call it an increased *braking effect* because either way, the car slowed, and hence, braked.

Falling in love can be from an increase in dopamine, a decrease in other chemicals, or perhaps both. We now think that the increase in dopamine effect in schizophrenia could be from a decrease in *glutamate*, another brain chemical that causes stimulation of brain activity. We all know of the old person who, as he ages, becomes suspicious, perhaps feels that somebody is stealing from him, and even starts to see people who aren't there. With aging, brain systems tend to weaken, not become stronger. So this increase in the dopamine effect could be from a decline in another chemical in the brain, such as glutamate. Here, the car is going slower because we're pushing on the accelerator with less force.

> *The point to make is that an increased dopamine effect could be caused by more dopamine or by a reduction in other, opposing chemicals.*

Let's look at what dopamine is and what it does in our brain, and get an idea of how it does what it does.

Dopamine is a neurotransmitter—a chemical substance that is released (transmitted) by one brain cell to send a signal to another brain cell. It's communication between two cells in the brain, just like us communicating with our neighbor with a casual across-the-street chat. But brain cell communication happens on an infinitely small level.

To understand how the chemicals of love work on our brain and change our perceptions, we need to review how brain cells communicate with each other.

In the simplest life form, if an organism has only one cell, there is no need for communication with other cells. In an organism with multiple cells, these cells need to communicate with each other to coordinate their activities.

Cells use the same communication mode that we use to communicate with our neighbor across the street.

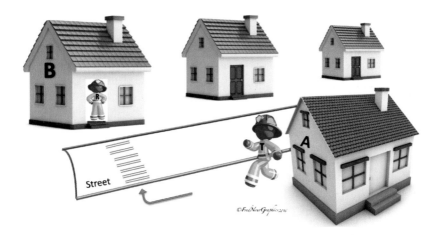

*Cell communication model*

In the diagram, House A wants House B to turn up their heat.

So how does House A communicate the request?

House A sends their son, Thomas, to cross the street and talk to his friend Robert, who happens to be standing outside House B. Hearing what Thomas has to say, Robert agrees to go inside the house and ask his parents to turn up the heat. House B is warmer now.

Thomas is the message carrier, the *transmitter* of the message.

Robert is the message receiver, or its *receptor*.

That's exactly how brain cells communicate with each other.

Since medical terminology is written in Latin, we'll translate this to medical Latin in the table on the next page.

| General English | Medical Latin |
| --- | --- |
| House | Cell |
| Street | Synapse |
| Thomas, the messenger | Transmitter, Thomas |
| Robert, the message receiver | Receptor, Robert |
| If Thomas carries the message in the brain | Neuro-transmitter Thomas |
| If Thomas carries the message in the blood | Hormone Thomas |

*All we need to understand here is that you need one cell to release the chemical, and a specialized structure to receive it. The first is the transmitter; the second is the receptor.*

## Where Is Dopamine Located in Our Brain?

The short answer: in more than one place. There are several dopamine systems in the brain. Each system deals with a different function. An analogy would be the various liquids in your car. Some are to cool the engine, and some help the brakes do their very important task; others keep the transmission shifting or help melt the ice off the windshield when the weather turns wet and frigid, and so on. These are all liquids, but they serve different functions in different systems. In a similar way, dopamine can stimulate us or calm us down. A patient with Parkinson's disease suffers from excess involuntary movements, like hand tremors; giving the patient dopamine (L-dopa) resolves the tremors. Here, dopamine is a calmer.

The Thomas-and-Robert example of dopamine transfer is very simple, but dopamine systems are extremely multifaceted, with many types of dopamine receptors, extensive networks of cell connections, and a myriad of effects on many other brain chemicals in a dynamic and tremendously complex way. The one reliable thing to say is that dopamine is used mainly in the intermediate limbic brain. The diagram to the right is just to show you how complex the dopamine system is, with multiple neurotransmitters interacting together continuously.

Thank goodness, all you really need to know is that dopamine control uses multiple, complex systems.

Dopamine is released by a network of cells. This is akin to the

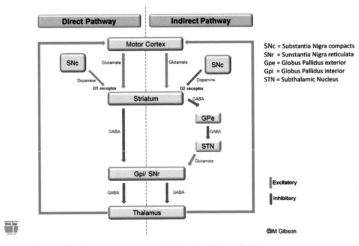

*Basal ganglia, dopamine networks in Parkinson's disease*

movement of the ball in football and soccer; movements aren't always in the same sequence. One of the players in this "dopamine game" is the *ventral tegmental area*, but this is just one location out of a complex network of cells. Though I don't share their belief, many nonmedical authors believe the ventral tegmental area is the brain's love center. The simple reason for my disagreement is that if love resides in this area, then a small stroke or cancer damaging the area would cause immediate loss of all the love we have, including our affection for those we currently love and have loved in the past. This doesn't happen. Also, inflammation or infection in or near the ventral tegmental area will stimulate it, and that should cause us to feel more intense love. Electrical deep-brain stimulation of this area doesn't change how we love others. Neither damage nor stimulation of the ventral tegmental area will change our feelings of love.

The ventral tegmental area is just one of the players in the game of love.

*The ventral tegmental area is not the "love center" in the brain.*

Adding to the kettle of complexity, there is dopamine in the bloodstream that has nothing to do with the brain dopamine. Dopamine in the brain has effects on hormones, and hormones affect dopamine as well.

Next, I'll briefly discuss how dopamine affects our behavior.

## Dopamine and Intermediate Limbic Brain Systems

Ah, yes, let's talk about dopamine and emotions. Dopamine is used in the reward systems for many behaviors, good and bad, as you've learned. It's involved in addiction, sex, love, euphoria, and much more.

The intermediate limbic brain, via dopamine release, causes us to feel extreme joy, pleasure, excitement, and happiness. Intermediate limbic brain memory, probably through norepinephrine, generates a drive to seek the rewards repeatedly. The problem with many of these functions isn't the dopamine but the brain's memory that remembers the reward from dopamine and seeks it repeatedly, until the desire becomes a compulsion—the desire to have the reward again and again, even against our will—or even an addiction.

Serotonin is involved in compulsions, as we'll learn about later, yet if you suddenly stop giving dopamine to someone, no harm to the body occurs. Or if we give someone too much dopamine, no serious harm to the body will happen. In addictions, though, the brain changes its response to the drugs, and the brain functioning changes permanently. Suddenly stopping the drugs could cause fatal withdrawal. An overdose of an addictive substance can be fatal. Giving dopamine to the drug addict doesn't fix the withdrawal problem. We never treat drug withdrawals by giving dopamine. Addictions are physiologically different from obsessions.

We have quite limited conscious control over dopamine-induced urges. If a person uses cocaine only once in their life, that person becomes a cocaine addict for the rest of their life. This is because cocaine causes a massive release of dopamine in the intermediate limbic brain. This release is what addicts call a "hit" from cocaine, and it's associated with an extreme sense of euphoria and joy. The memory of that experience will be permanently stored in the intermediate limbic brain, never to be erased. The reward itself is short-lived, yet the memory of the reward is permanent. After a single use, the person is now addicted to cocaine, and his or her brain will keep demanding a recurrence of that feeling of euphoria, demanding the release of dopamine again, in effect demanding more cocaine.

Gamblers have the same disease process when gambling. The sudden winning of a large sum of money creates an equally sudden, massive release of dopamine associated with an extreme sense of joy and happiness.

The memory of that dopamine-release feeling will stay in the intermediate limbic brain. The gambler will have the intense urge to pursue this dopamine surge again and will spend a lifetime trying to fight that urge. There is no need to mention that many lives have been ruined by a gambling compulsion.

Compulsive shoppers have the same problem. Dopamine is released in their brains when they buy something new, and they get excited about the purchases. Experiencing joy, happiness, and excitement, they daydream about how attractive they look in these new purchases, how others will be impressed by their new acquisitions, and so on. These good feelings are from the dopamine effect. The memory system learns that shopping caused that feeling by releasing dopamine, and desires it again and again, regardless of the lives destroyed by accumulated credit card debts they can never pay back. The compulsive knows he or she should stop shopping but can't resist the urge, the desire to release that dopamine again.

*Dopamine release induces a motivation to acquire a reward.*

The intermediate limbic brain learns through epinephrine and norepinephrine, and never forgets.

Orgasm is caused by dopamine release. The dopamine-release experience induces a motivation to acquire the reward repeatedly. In some susceptible individuals, this can cause a problematic hypersexuality compulsion.

But remember, there are dopamine receptors as well as dopamine transmitters. Dopamine can be a stimulator or an inhibitor of the brain. We have five different types of dopamine receptors, termed as "D1" to "D5." Each type has a different effect on the brain. For example, D2 stimulation by dopamine induces different behaviors and feelings for which no memory is stored and there is no desire to seek its release again. The best example is nausea and vomiting. D2 stimulation causes the nausea, and if the stimulation is more severe, vomiting. D2 receptor blockers stop the nausea and vomiting, leaving absolutely no desire to experience more nausea and vomiting. This is different from D1 stimulation, which enhances addiction.

*The point is that not all dopamine receptors cause addiction or compulsion—only some of them do so.*

Can we actually artificially create these behaviors in people?

Yes, we can.

Parkinson's disease is caused by a decrease in dopamine's effect, so it is treated with the dopamine precursor L-dopa, and/or other dopamine-increasing medications.

Neurologists learned that certain susceptible individuals might start to have many of these nonmovement-related behaviors. If we give too much dopamine, a patient might spend an entire fortune on gambling or shopping. Some suddenly become hypersexual. Some have tried risky behaviors such as jumping from a cliff into the sea. This is very rare but has happened. The susceptibility to these behaviors is based on a genetic variation in a gene called *tryptophan hydroxylase type 2*. The most interesting thing about this gene is that it has no effect on dopamine at all; the gene works on serotonin. This raises the question: Are addictions a serotonin problem? More research is being done now on this interesting finding.

These people are already at risk of these dopamine-induced behaviors before we start to increase their brain's dopamine effect. Some patients become paranoid. Hallucinations, in fact, are the most common manifestation of a high dopamine dose. When we reduce the dopamine dose or switch them from dopamine-increasing medications to other, non-dopamine medications, these abnormal behaviors disappear, and the patients return to their normal behavior.

• • •

Shakespeare compared love to madness, but to most, it's a most delicious madness. You'll likely recognize the lyrics to this song sung by Celine Dion, one that nicely illustrates the waiting for love, then the effects of falling in love: romantic love.

A New Day Has Come
*I was waiting for so long*
*For a miracle to come*
*Everyone told me to be strong*
*Hold on and don't shed a tear*

*So through darkness and good times*
*I knew I'd make it through*
*And the world thought I had it all*
*But I was waiting for you*

*Hush now*
*I see a light in the sky*
*Oh it's almost blinding me*
*I can't believe I've been touched by an angel*
*With love*
*Let the rain come down*
*And wash away my tears*
*Let it fill my soul*
*And drown my fears*
*Let it shatter the walls*
*For a new sun*

*A new day has come*
*Where it was dark now there is light*
*Where there was pain, now there's joy*
*Where there was weakness, I found my strength*
*All in the eyes of a boy*
*Let it shatter the walls*
*For a new sun*
*A new day has come.*

In this song, Dion compares the heady rush and other sweeping sensations and emotions to the dawning of a new and glorious day, telling the story of someone who has had their entire world upended by falling in love. And yes, within the brain, it's a lot like that, too.

We've all heard that love is blind. But why is it blind? What makes us fail to see reality when we're in love? There's a physical basis for this, in where and how it happens. To understand how love alters our perceptions, let's briefly review the "relay stations" for sensations in the brain.

First we'll look at our current sensory system and at how our current sensory system evolved. It all begins with three little nerves.

The old reptilian brain has sensory nerves going to it. The one illustrated in red is called the *first-order sensory neuron*. This nerve carries sensations from the skin to the old reptilian brain.

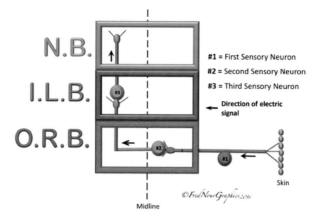

*Basic sensory nerves*

With the addition of the intermediate limbic brain, a second nerve was added: the *second-order neuron* (illustrated in green). This nerve starts in the old reptilian brain and ends in the intermediate limbic brain.

This development added an effect for emotions on perceptions. Now the animal can feel fear upon perceiving certain information, such as a gazelle spotting a nearby cheetah. The gazelle will have a more intense response to the threat than the one provided by the old reptilian brain alone, although the old reptilian brain will still cause the heart to beat faster and stronger, with more blood pumped to the muscles to run faster, and so on.

The new brain hasn't evolved yet, of course, so it has no connections down to the intermediate limbic brain. We can't consciously change the fear reaction.

*The intermediate limbic brain adds emotional dimension to sensory perceptions.*

With the addition of the new brain, a third nerve was added: the *third-order neuron*. That one is illustrated in blue on the chart. This third-order nerve starts in the intermediate limbic brain and ends in the new brain. This is the nerve responsible for consciously feeling your body sensations, such as pain, numbness, and tingling.

*The new brain adds conscious awareness of sensory perceptions.*

Taken altogether, it's now time to dig in and find out how those three little nerves work together in a romantic way.

• • •

When we're in, it's the intermediate limbic brain changes the message, because the intermediate limbic brain is the middleman in the transmission of the message.

An analogy:

CIA agents collect information about the nation. These are the *first-order persons.*

Information collected is given to the director of the CIA—the *second-order person.*

The CIA director gives the information to the president. This is the *third-order person.*

Now, if a CIA agent finds out there was an explosion that killed twenty people, he will transmit the information to the CIA director. If the CIA director transmits it to the president as an explosion that killed twenty people, the president will believe there was an explosion that killed twenty people, and will act accordingly.

Now, if the CIA director changes the message to something like, "There was an explosion that killed two thousand people," the president will believe that *two thousand people*, not twenty, were killed in an explosion. His reaction will be quite different. Or, if the CIA director changed the message to "There were no explosions at all," the president, quite reasonably, won't react at all.

In other words, the second-order person can alter the president's perception of reality. The president has no way of knowing the message was altered. He believes that the CIA agent sent the message of two thousand people killed in an explosion, or that there were no explosions at all.

As the signal gets to the new brain using its relay station in the intermediate limbic brain, it can make the conscious brain perceive sensations as more intense, or less intense, by enhancing or blocking the release of a neurotransmitter, or by enhancing or blocking the receptor's response to the neurotransmitter. There is little conscious control over this modulation of sensations. Like the president, the new brain completely believes everything it receives from the intermediate limbic brain. It can't tell whether the information has been modified by the intermediate limbic brain.

*The intermediate limbic brain modifies our conscious perception of sensations based on our emotions. We have no conscious control over this modulation.*

It should be noted that the old reptilian brain in reptiles is very similar to the old reptilian brain in birds (birds have the same old reptilian brain, but with the addition of the newer intermediate limbic brain). Humans have the same old reptilian brain that reptiles and birds have, and the same intermediate limbic brain that birds have, but we have the newest addition, the new brain. We keep adding to the oldest brain with newer abilities, but we keep the old abilities as they are. Only the new brain is different in humans.

## Human Examples of Excess Monoamines Effects on the Brain

You will learn a lot more about transmitters and receptors now and have a definite idea of how human brains differ from all other animal brains on the planet. Now, back to the catecholamines: epinephrine, norepinephrine, and dopamine as well as serotonin, that all-important team of chemicals when it comes to love.

If I claim that some feature of falling in love is caused by the excess effects of monoamines, then we should see some similar manifestations in brain disorders caused by an excess monoamines effect.

Let's look at a disease that's associated with excess monoamines effect, in fact the most common disease that's in part related to increased monoamine effects: schizophrenia. In these patients, the excess monoamines effect causes a change in perception and behavior, among other features, that's similar to the example of the CIA agent, CIA director, and president, where the CIA director changes the information and thus changes the president's perception of events.

If we look at the symptoms caused by the excess monoamines effect in schizophrenics, then some symptoms of falling in love could be similar to the manifestations seen in this disease.

*Could this be what Shakespeare was referring to when he
said "Love is merely a madness"?*

Here are some of the common manifestations of increased mono-amines effects as seen in schizophrenia.

## Hoarding

The perception with hoarding is that every tiny little thing is so important and must be preserved. These sufferers have a household full of "junk" that they firmly believe is vitally important and valuable. "One day, this will be worth millions of dollars" is a typical statement. Hoarding is a form of compulsion. These items usually cause the hoarder a special joy from looking back at them and recalling certain memories associated with the items. Compulsions are driven by serotonin. The joy in the memory is induced by the epinephrine effect on the intermediate limbic brain.

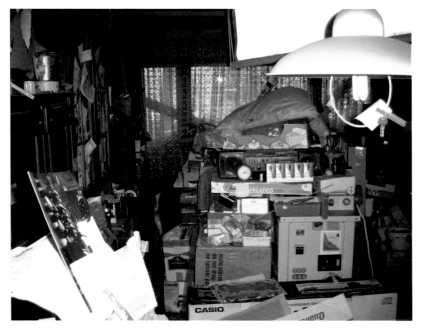

*Hoarding*

*Illusion*

A stimulus is an item that provokes a signal to the brain. An image seen by the eye, a sound heard by the ear, or a touch on the skin are all examples of a stimuli. Illusion is an altered perception of a *real* stimulus. The signal is transmitted to the new brain via three nerves, one in each segment of the brain. An example of illusion is the misinterpreted hearing of a chirping bird. That chirping sound signals in its way through the brain, but—most likely in the intermediate limbic brain—it's changed by monoamine, so the conscious brain will perceive it as, for example, a song, not just a chirp. The person might perceive the sound as if the bird is actually singing love songs to them. The new brain perceives the sound sensation, which isn't the same original sensation, but the brain always believes that what it receives is "the truth, the whole truth, and nothing but the truth," so that person becomes convinced that "The bird is singing love songs to me." There is no way you can consciously convince them otherwise. Yet, if we block the excess monoamine effects, probably in the intermediate limbic brain, the chirps are now perceived as just bird chirps, not as a love song.

Another example of illusion is seeing a photo of someone and perceiving that the person in the photo is someone else—for example, a famous person. A picture of one's brother might be believed to be of Jesus.

*Delusions*

Delusions are fixed false beliefs or feelings. The belief has no basis in reality, but there's no way to change that perception consciously, no matter how hard or how long you try; hence, these delusions are called "fixed." The person suffering a delusion usually has a false belief about himself or herself. They can feel they are a genius and know everything about everything—an example of a grandiose delusion. It's that feeling a schizophrenic person has that he's a famous person, such as Albert Einstein or Napoleon Bonaparte. He isn't, but you can never convince him otherwise.

Some sufferers can have paranoid delusions, an exaggerated fear about another person. A dramatic example is the person who has the fixed belief that his neighbor is trying to poison him or have him killed, or that the guy sitting across from him in the doctor's waiting room is a Russian spy trying to murder him. Again, if we manipulate monoamines, these beliefs can disappear or be reduced significantly. Delusions, like illusions, are believed to be dopamine driven.

## Jealousy

This is a form of fear or paranoia caused by epinephrine release. In jealousy, the perception of a threat far exceeds the reality. It's seen in both sexes, but is thought to be more intense in females than males. This is believed to be a manifestation of the female unconscious awareness of the fewer eggs they have and the desire to avoid losing any eggs waiting for another mate. One study that seems to support this concerned jealousy in rats. They had a female rat mate with a male rat few times. Then they introduced a new estrus (in-heat) female rat into the cage. I was surprised to learn how violent and aggressive the original female rat was toward the new female rat, to the point of attempting to literally kill the new female rat.

## Unclear or Confused Thinking

Those suffering this symptom can't make logical conclusions for obviously simple problems. It's ninety degrees outside, and they want to go to the beach. They put on their heaviest sweater and thick gloves and wear the long boots. They go to a job interview wearing their flip-flops, fur hat, and pajamas. This is believed to be dopamine induced.

## Obsession

Repeatedly thinking about the same topic or subject is involuntary and can't be stopped consciously. The sufferer wants to consciously think about something else (new brain), but simply can't; the subconscious urge to think about that topic keeps intruding into their conscious mind. These are called intrusive obsessions. Obsessions are serotonin related.

## Compulsion

This is the irresistible urge to do certain things against one's will. The sufferer doesn't want to do it but simply can't resist the urge. The typical example is the person who keeps washing his hands repeatedly until the skin ulcerates, but he still can't stop doing it. Gambling is similar in its chemical basis in the brain. The gambler can't stop himself from going to the casino with his money. Compulsive shopping has the same chemical basis. Risky behavior is the urge to do things the person knows are dangerous but can't stop the urge to do it. An example is jumping from the second-floor balcony into a swimming pool. All these urges are from serotonin effects.

*Euphoria*

This is the sense of extreme joy, happiness, and near ecstasy, to the point where the person is walking about singing or laughing at nothing. They keep talking and giggling to themselves. There's no reason for this joy; if you ask, they don't know why they're so happy. Euphoria is dopamine related.

What does all this have to do with love?

If falling in love is caused by an excess monoamines effect, then we can have similar or related symptoms to schizophrenia when we fall in love.

You might be asking, "Is that true? Can we really act like a mild schizophrenic when we fall in love?"

The answer isn't *quite* a yes or no, so we'll discuss that in the next chapter, when we talk about the romantic love phase of love.

## Evidence That Monoamines Are Absolutely or Relatively Increased in the Early Stages of Love

Not only schizophrenia but the clinical manifestations of falling in love match the same clinical manifestations of other disorders known to be caused by relative excess of monoamines in the brain.

Many animal studies proved the increased effect of dopamine with mating, when the researchers increased and blocked dopamine in different ways to prove that it's involved with strong pair-bonding in voles (field mice). Repeated studies proved that increased dopamine effect is associated with attraction to the other sex. The most convincing evidence came in monogamous prairie voles (field mice); when a female mated with a male, she afterward became strongly bonded to him. If a dopamine agonist (an agonist increases the dopamine effect) was injected in the intermediate limbic brain system of a virgin female prairie vole, she bonded with a new nearby male even though she didn't copulate with him.

You'll see this adorable furry creature again, in a later chapter, and read about other contributions voles have made to our understanding of the brain and love.

In keeping with these studies, electrochemical studies on the intermediate limbic brain system of male rats proved the release of more dopamine in the intermediate limbic brain when the rat sees a receptive estrus (in-heat) female rat. Dopamine stimulates the sex drive by acting on the sexual dimorphic nucleus.

Note: If the discussion of animal studies makes you squeamish, be soothed by the fact that many studies were also done on humans, who were willing to take risks for the sake of advancing science, or often, in the desperate hope of being cured of some malady not helped by other measures.

Common experience and social studies suggest that this excess monoamines period lasts for about two years on average, then fades away. This could suggest that in the early stages of love, there are increased monoamine effects in the monoamine-rich intermediate limbic brain centers that gradually fade away as love gets older, usually in about twenty-four months, plus or minus a few months.

These studies show that there is some physical evidence that the increased monoamine effect is associated with the early stages of love and that this increase fades after a period of time.

Now we're done with the first "child" in the monoamines family, the catecholamines, with its three children, epinephrine, norepinephrine, and dopamine. Let's move to the other child in the monoamines family, serotonin.

## Serotonin

Serotonin is another brain neurotransmitter, the last member of the monoamines family and the brother of the catecholamines. Serotonin is present in many body systems: the blood, the guts, and the brain. Only ten percent of the body's serotonin is in the brain.

Below, you'll find out how serotonin modulates (affects) other brain systems. You'll also see how serotonin affects the falling-in-love phase by affecting dopamine and norepinephrine and how serotonin affects nonapeptides responsible for phase four of love, True Love. We'll see how serotonin affects our appetite, sex drive, and sleep and how serotonin enhances the memory of falling in love. We will learn how serotonin suppresses hallucinations and compulsions. While you might think that at least a few of these couldn't be related to love, rest assured, *all* these are part of the love phases.

Serotonin-making cells are located in the brain in a location called the *raphe* nucleus. *Raphe* is a Greek word that means "seam." The raphe nucleus is in the midline of the old reptilian brain, as if it's in the seam between the right and left halves of the brain.

Many serotonin receptors perform different functions, and are termed serotonin receptor type 1 through type 7. Some receptors have subtypes, such as serotonin receptor type 1, which has subtype 1A, 1B, 1D, 1E, and 1F. (There was once a 1C, but it was discovered to be unrelated to serotonin and was removed.)

Different types of serotonin receptors affect the brain differently, sometimes in opposing ways. More serotonin at one receptor can cause a certain effect, while more serotonin at another receptor can cause the opposite effect. This is like the example I gave just a bit ago, where more pressure on the acceleration pedal or the brake pedal causes different effects. We can't reliably say "increased (or decreased) serotonin can do this or that." It all depends on which receptor is stimulated (more effect) or suppressed (less effect).

Serotonin receptor 1A stimulation enhances memory and learning, reduces anxiety and depression, reduces pain, prevents migraines, and reduces aggression. If you stimulate 1A receptors you release dopamine in your prefrontal cortex, causing you to feel more intense falling-in-love feelings. Some nonmedical authors believe that increasing serotonin levels reduces dopamine levels, impairing the feelings of falling in love. But think about that. Have you ever heard of someone who was in such an intense romantic love because their serotonin levels went so low from severe depression? In effect, saying, "I love more intensely when depressed than when I'm happy?" Of course not.

If you stimulate serotonin receptor 2A, you release more norepinephrine and glutamates (another brain neurotransmitter). Both enhance the feeling of love, as mentioned earlier.

Serotonin receptor 2C releases dopamine, causing an increase in appetite. Interestingly, stimulation of this receptor *induces* depression, so this has the opposite effect of stimulation of serotonin receptor 1A, which *reduces* depression.

If you stimulate serotonin receptor 3, you vomit.

There is evidence for direct connection of serotonin cells on the VTA (ventral tegmental area) dopamine cells. One effect of dopamine increase from more serotonin effect is increased appetite, which is the cause of weight gain seen with some antidepressants. This was proven by deep brain stimulation of the VTA.

The decrease of serotonin stimulation on the VTA seen in depression causes a decrease on dopamine effects on the sexually dimorphic nucleus (SDN) in the hypothalamus. The decrease in sex drive seen in depressed patients is caused by this decrease in dopamine effect.

Serotonin is known to have a connection with the nonapeptides oxytocin and vasopressin. Serotonin stimulation causes an increased release of oxytocin, one of the True Love chemicals that causes increased bonding.

*Serotonin works indirectly to enhance True Love by increasing dopamine, norepinephrine, and nonapeptides.*

Most serotonin is recycled by taking back (reuptake), which puts it back in the cells. Serotonin is a very durable chemical, which makes the rate of making new serotonin slow, and the system doesn't need to make much new serotonin. That's why serotonin-enhancing medications are slow to work.

There are many myths about treatment with serotonin. The worst myth is that it's effective only for depression, and if a person doesn't feel depressed, they shouldn't take serotonin-enhancing medication.

This is completely false. Saying that antidepressants are "just for depression" is like saying that aspirin is "just for headaches." Should people who are at risk of strokes and heart attacks, or who have a fever but don't have headaches, not take aspirin, when there is overwhelming evidence that small-dose aspirin can save lives and aspirin can relieve a fever? That would be lunacy.

We physicians use serotonin to treat depression, of course. But, in undepressed patients, we also use it to potentially cure memory problems in a neurological disease called *pseudo-dementia*. We use serotonin enhancers to prevent bedwetting in children who aren't depressed at all. All of us use serotonin to maintain sleep. We start sleep with a brain neurotransmitter called *GABA*, and stay asleep with serotonin, akin to the

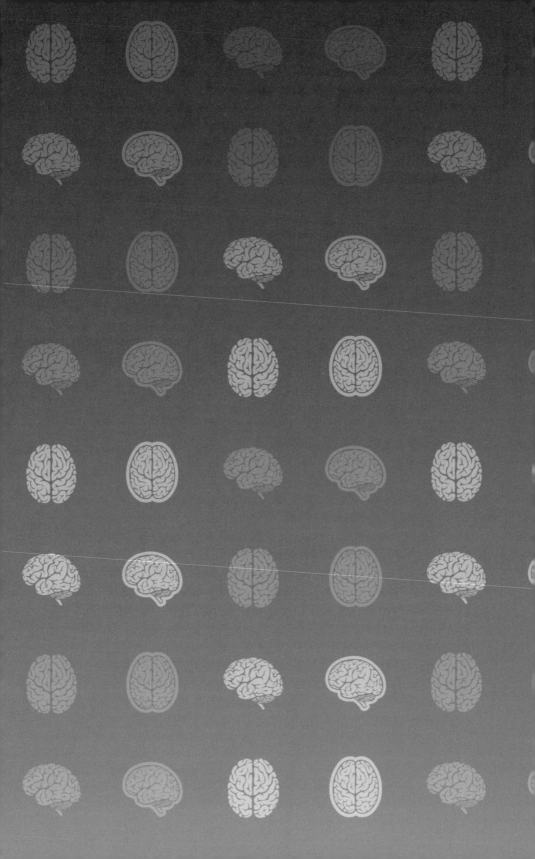

## CHAPTER 7

# PHASE TWO OF LOVE—
# ROMANTIC LOVE/FALLING IN LOVE

---

Do you remember this song, sung long ago by a fellow named Frank?

*Strangers in the night exchanging glances*
*Wondering in the night what were the chances*
*We'd be sharing love before the night was through*
*Something in your eyes was so inviting*
*Something in your smile was so exciting*
*Something in my heart told me I must have you*
*Strangers in the night*
*Two lonely people, we were strangers in the night*
*Up to the moment when we said our first hello, little did we know*
*Love was just a glance away, a warm embracing dance away*
*and*
*Ever since that night, we've been together*
*Lovers at first sight, in love forever*
*It turned out so right for strangers in the night.*

Two perfect strangers exchange glances, have "a warm embracing dance," and voila, they are in love forever!

This is love as most of us perceive it, meeting someone and then instantaneously feeling the wonderful feeling of love "forever." We all dream and wish for this to happen to us one day.

We call this *romantic love, sexual love, passionate love, warm love,* just *love* or *falling in love.*

Why do we call it *falling?*

It's because falling happens suddenly, forcefully, effortlessly, and unexpectedly. We have no power to stop or change the fall. We just accept that the fall happened, and we just have to accept the outcome of the fall.

Why do we call it *falling in love?*

It's because falling in love happens suddenly, forcefully, effortlessly, and unexpectedly. We have no power to stop the falling in love, or change the result. We just accept that falling in love happened and that we have to accept the outcome of falling in love since our conscious brain (new brain) can't totally stop or change what happens in our intermediate limbic brain.

How does this phase of love happen?

Falling in love can happen suddenly, or it could take a short while to fully develop. It seems that those who have a powerful intermediate limbic brain and weak new brain fall in love quickly. The new brain takes a longer time to analyze the mate's worthiness. The intermediate limbic brain is instinctual and quick. Or, those who have a strong new brain influence, with a stronger norepinephrine system, use it to consciously and cognitively, if slowly, make a selection. The latter approach still uses the intermediate limbic brain, of course, or there would be no love feelings.

## Sudden Falling in Love

When I myself first fell in love, I perceived love subjectively, looking from the inside out. I couldn't see myself. I could not recognize what was happening to me or how it happened.

I recall going to do rounds at my hospital. As I entered my patients' ward, my eyes fell on a young physical therapist sitting down, reading my notes on a patient of mine. I recall thinking immediately that this was the woman I'd been dreaming of all my life. That I must get her attention. On legs I was no longer certain belonged to me, I went over and asked her, "Why are you reading my notes without my permission?" I gave her my pager number and instructed her to call me every time she was going to read one of my notes.

Obviously, she got the message. The rest is the usual series of events. I only knew that I felt wonderful, full of joy and pleasure. I never felt any changes in me or in my brain.

Many years later, I had the chance to see the "falling" part of falling in love objectively. I saw it in a totally different light this time.

Back when I was a first-year resident in neurology, we had a regular morning meeting with a teaching faculty member to discuss the new patients admitted the night before. We called this the morning report. Afterward, all residents met to distribute the new patients among ourselves based on the existing patient load we each had that day. A few residents would first go to attend to urgent patient needs that had been deferred during the faculty morning report or held over from the previous night. While waiting for their return, the rest of us had a few minutes to chitchat until everybody was back to the residents' room.

Rotating with me at the same hospital was Nicole, who I introduced earlier. I saw Nicole every morning during the morning report if neither of us had been called away for something urgent, and I enjoyed our morning chats.

One morning Nicole came in with an unusually big smile on her face, and I had to ask her, "Nicole, what happened to you? I've never seen you look so elated."

"That's because I'm in love."

At first I thought she was joking, so I chuckled. "Just like that? Yesterday you were perfectly normal, and today you're suddenly in love?"

"Yesterday I hadn't met Brandon. Today I've already met Brandon. I feel wonderful because I love Brandon."

I was incredulous, but it slowly dawned on me that she might be serious. "Wow, just like that and you're in love!"

"Yes. Just like that. I know my heart very well!"

*How did* that *happen?* I wondered. And of course I had to ask.

"Yesterday I was at a friend's house, at a party," she said. "I opened the door, and my eyes fell on Brandon. I knew immediately that he's the man of my dreams. He glanced at me too, and," she sighed, "his face just lit up. I maneuvered my way toward him, and he did the same. We talked a little while, and that was it. I'm in love with him!"

I worked hard to hide my disbelief, and said, "Nicole, what do you know about Brandon?"

"He is just a *wonderful* man who's in love with me. That's all I need to know. That's all that matters."

Quietly shocked at how quickly this happened but also curious, I kept an ear out for her, hoping this was an infatuation and would soon burn itself out. But as days, then weeks of morning chats went by, her glowing enthusiasm for her new love didn't waver.

A month later was the neurology department's annual holiday party. By tradition, everyone was expected in the reception hall with any of our significant others. Nicole was there, looking attractive and glamorous, together with her Brandon. Wanting to observe her before she spotted me, I partly hid myself beside the entrance, where there were some dusty-looking artificial trees.

A few minutes later, another neurology resident you've met before, John, came to me looking agitated and said, "I can't believe it. I just can't believe that Nicole's dating this guy!"

"Why?" I said, trying not to sneeze.

"I went up to them to say hello, and I asked him, 'Brandon, what college did you go to?' He said, 'Oh, I didn't need college, just graduated high school.' Can you believe that?"

That did seem more than a little implausible. Like the rest of us, Nicole started her education with a college degree and then four years of med school followed by a four-year residency—hers in pediatrics. But she'd gone further and was doing a two-year fellowship in neurology with us. I said all I could say: "Well, John, they say love is blind. Look at his big muscles, his big body. He's also really handsome. Maybe he has a successful business or is some big artist?"

John shook his head, dislodging another raft of dust from the plant. "No, he's not. I asked him what kind of work he's in. He told me he's a warehouse manager."

I grasped John's arm, and together we moved away from the plant. "Wow, that *is* shocking," I said. "I don't know if it will do any good, but maybe we can help her see the big picture. Let's talk to her tomorrow after morning report."

John and I waited until after morning report to ask Nicole to hang out with us in front of the building. Still clearly buoyant in mood, she gave us curious looks but agreed.

John didn't speak up, which left it to me to start. "Ah, Nicole," I began, "we have no business delving into your love life. You know we both care a lot about you. But we're very … concerned … about you."

Her expression now showed confusion. "Why is that?"

At last, John found his voice. "Nicole, think about it. You're highly educated, intelligent. No, you're brilliant! We just feel this guy isn't a good match for you. That you're making a mistake—"

Nicole's shocked gasp stopped him. She blurted, "It doesn't matter what kind of education he has, or what job he can do, how intelligent or unintelligent he is. The only thing that matters is that we're in love with each other. Nothing else on earth matters more. I know that—" She bit her lip, but then continued. "Love will change everything from now on. Don't worry about me. I'm extremely happy with him. Haven't you heard the saying 'Love conquers all'?"

We had, of course, and what do you say to that? Wondering why she'd hesitated but uncomfortable asking, I mumbled some apology and took John's arm and we headed back inside, John a bit less willingly than I.

A few months later, John came to me again, this time more agitated. "You won't believe what I just found out about Nicole's guy," he said the moment we were alone.

In truth, I had decided to live and let live about Nicole's situation, but John hadn't. "What did you find out?" I said.

"You probably noticed how down she looked at morning meeting."

"I did, but I thought maybe she just had a late night."

John shook his head. "Nope. While we were walking across the bridge after the meeting, I asked her what was the matter. She told me that Brandon lost his job. She believes that another guy didn't like Brandon and backstabbed him to get his position. I asked her what this other man did to get Brandon's job … Fred, you'll never believe what she told me … the other guy told their boss about Brandon's criminal record. Yes, she knew that Brandon has a criminal record!"

"Oh my God," I managed. "She is insane. I don't understand at all … how *can't* she see all the problems she's getting herself into?"

"Yeah. I mean, how she can diagnose the most difficult and complex cases with extreme ease and perfect judgment and not see how screwed-up this is? How can she be totally unable to see that Brandon's just not the right guy for her? She must have a focal psychosis."

"Focal" means "localized," and "psychosis" is the name for a group of thought disorders such as schizophrenia. In effect, John thought our dear friend was crazy for sticking with a man so obviously wrong for her.

Hearing what I'd just heard, I couldn't say I disagreed.

I drew in a breath, then blew it out slowly, trying to think. "Maybe this time she'll listen to us, start to see the reality of what's going on. We have to try."

We managed to locate Nicole before our workdays ended.

This time, I didn't wait for John. "Nicole, I'm so sorry, but I just can't have any finesse dealing with this. We both believe you're going psychotic. Look at it from our perspective—you know this guy has a criminal record and you're still in love with him? Sorry, but this is totally insane!"

Shoulders straight, chin set, she said, "The ... crimes happened before he fell in love with me. Now things have completely changed. That was in the past and has absolutely no effect on us today, or on our future. Everything's totally different now."

She stopped speaking but turned her gaze from me to John, then back. "You two aren't in love. You'll understand when you both experience something so life changing." She gave smiles meant to reassure us and squeezed John's arm, then mine. "Don't worry about me. Just go and look for your own love!"

Her reassurance didn't change my thinking. I remained fearful about what seemed to be happening to her neuro-physiologically (in her brain function) and worried about her as my friend. I'd studied the brain in detail but didn't have a good explanation for this. I'd been partly bluffing before, but *did* she have a brain disorder I didn't know about?

More questions came: *Why can't she see the guy for who he is? People keep telling me this is typical of love, that love's blind. But why is it blind? Why on earth would we have this insanity called love? Perhaps William Shakespeare was correct to say that love is merely madness.*

In the end, I realized that Nicole had predominantly used her intermediate limbic brain to make a mate selection. We continued to have our chats, but I kept my concerns to myself, reminding myself that she was my friend, not a potential patient. There was no need to engage my new brain in wasting time with further analysis of the suitability of her chosen mate. The intermediate limbic brain made the decision, and we would all have to accept her choice. The distractions of school and work kept my worries in the background most of the time.

## Gradual Falling in Love

Let's look at the story of the movie *The English Patient*.

Almásy is a Hungarian cartographer. In the late 1930s, he is exploring and mapping the North African desert with Peter Maddox, the expedition's leader. Their expedition is joined by a British couple, Geoffrey and Katherine Clifton. Katherine doesn't really notice Almásy until he follows her while she's at the old market in Cairo. Her interest in him peaks when she accidentally discovers in his personal notebook that he's writing notes about her beauty and charm. Sensing he's in love with her, she starts to pay attention to his worthiness. While Peter Maddox is away, getting more supplies, she falls in love with Almásy. The rest of the story is about the emotions of falling in love.

Katherine didn't react like Nicole and fall in love at first sight. Katherine used her new brain to study her potential mate, taking her time to analyze and understand him before she engaged her intermediate limbic brain. It took her longer to make a mate selection.

Yet by all appearances, their love was as strong as the love between Nicole and Brandon.

Based on what scientists have learned so far, here's my explanation of what happens in this phase of love.

As we discussed before, we first build an image of the person of our dreams. This image, our fantasia, is stored in our intermediate limbic brain. It's like a template stored in our brain computer. Another component of our fantasia is stored in the intermediate limbic brain from decisions by the new brain to help in the conscious process of mate selection.

To understand what happens when we meet that special Person of My Dreams, let's look at an analogy. In the early days of computers, I had an IBM computer that used DOS as its operating system. The hard drive had a whopping 20 megabytes of storage. Hard drives were physically large and noisy in those days. You could actually hear the hard drive when it loaded the RAM with bits and bytes of magnetic information. I was fascinated by the fact that if I went to the C prompt: "C:\" and just typed one letter, for example, the letter Q, then hit enter, I could hear the hard drive sending massive amounts of bytes to the computer RAM, a sound that kept going and going, and in a few minutes (yes, minutes!), the computer screen displayed the program "Quicken," loaded and ready for use.

Just one letter started an onslaught of bytes to the RAM. If you typed two letters: "QB," you heard a massive flow of bytes from the hard drive and finally saw on your monitor, "QuickBooks."

You just needed one or two letters, and suddenly and effortlessly the data kept flowing, and it kept going until it was finished. Once started, you couldn't stop it.

Likewise, in falling in love, we can't stop the massive, continuous flow of data after it starts. We must satisfy both the intermediate limbic brain and the new brain's fantasia, and when we see a mate who closely resembles the Person of My Dreams fantasia we fall in love, often as quickly as Nicole did. We feel highly impressed and fascinated by their skills, abilities, and talents (new brain), as well as their beauty and sex appeal (intermediate limbic brain). We now perceive them as perfect. Medically, this is called "idealization of our mate"—we change our perception of our mate so it matches exactly the template of our fantasia stored in the intermediate limbic brain memory.

Upon this attraction, this so-called chemistry, a sudden, unexpected, forceful, effortless, unstoppable flow of data starts to load in our intermediate limbic brain, just like the computer example above. This flow of data results in sudden, massive release of catecholamines in our intermediate limbic brain system. The reward-system neurotransmitter dopamine causes us to feel all the wonderful things we experience when we fall in love. Norepinephrine will give us the loss of sleep, the fast heartbeats, the dilated eyes, and the sweating. It will make us more attentive to our beloved mate and focus all our energy on that mate while ignoring everybody else (even, in Nicole's case, two concerned friends). Epinephrine will give us fear, jealousy, and suspicion but will also solidify our memories of falling in love. Serotonin will modulate all these activities.

"Falling in love" is the phase that inspired the writing of most of the love stories, most of the famous love songs, and most of the famous love poems. Most love stories discuss how two mates met (mate selection) and how they eventually fell in love. Almost all of them stop at that phase, making us believe that this feeling will last forever.

Just like the monoamines effect in schizophrenia, when we fall in love we probably release a massive amount of dopamine, epinephrine, norepinephrine, and serotonin; thus, we acquire some features of schizophrenia such as the following.

*Euphoria*: Extreme sense of joy and happiness. (I'm so happy because I'm in love!) Euphoria is dopamine induced.

*Hoarding*: Suddenly every little note or gift given to us by the beloved feels incredibly important and causes excess joy. We save each one for a lifetime. The strong memories of the feeling associated with these gifts are permanently stored in our intermediate limbic brain system, never to be forgotten. These feelings are always associated with these items. A guy told me he'd saved a plastic cup with his lover's lipstick for a few years. When the plastic started to disintegrate, he realized it was just a piece of plastic, which he could now throw away. Hoarding is serotonin induced.

*Sensations*: All our sensations are relayed in the intermediate limbic brain system. There, each one can be altered. The smell of the beloved is so exciting. The beloved looks exceptionally handsome or beautiful. The beloved's touch seems so sensuous. Their kiss is so sweet. The sound of their voice is so sexy, erotic. All the music and songs heard together are so beautiful. Even sitting on a swing together is so relaxing.

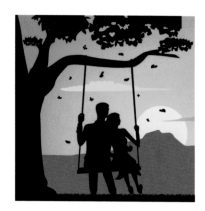

*Swinging together*

The visual image of the beloved is changed by the second-order neuron (the CIA director in examples earlier) in the intermediate limbic brain system to be perceived as the most beautiful images ever. The sky is now bluer, the trees are greener, and so on. Changes in sensory perceptions are dopamine induced.

*Illusions*: All sensations can be perceived in an idealized fashion. The sound isn't just so much more beautiful; it's actual songs. I have a story I'll discuss just a bit later about the sound of the word "Maria," and how beautiful this word could feel in her beloved's ears. For now, it's enough to know that illusions, too, are dopamine induced.

*Obsessions*: We continuously think about the beloved. The thoughts keep intruding on our normal thinking, and we can't stop them. This is called intrusive obsessive thinking, and is part of obsessive-compulsive disorder. Obsessions are the "thinking" component of the obsessive-compulsive disorder and are serotonin induced.

*Compulsions*: This is an irresistible urge to do certain things that we do almost against our will. Take, for example, the lover who writes four or five long love letters to his beloved every single day. The lover can't force him/herself to wait until the beloved writes back. Like the person who can't stop washing their hands, the letter-writing compulsion is the motor (physical action) component of obsessive-compulsive disorder. Compulsions are serotonin induced.

*Delusions*: Nicole believed that love would change Brandon, and she was totally and unshakably convinced that he would be a different man with love. That is a fixed (no one can convince her otherwise) and a false (he will never change) belief. This is a delusion. This is dopamine induced.

*Jealousy and paranoia*: We start to feel threatened by competing mates. We start to feel jealous about the beloved. We want to protect our love. Most of the time, this need to protect is perceived from unreasonable sources. I see no need for examples of jealousy; we all know a few stories of jealousy. This is a form of paranoid delusion and is epinephrine induced.

*Illogical thinking*: We start to have bizarre and unreasonable logic and unclear thinking. This is well illustrated in my experience with Nicole. She had perfect logic with brilliant thinking when she used her new brain to analyze complicated, intellectually challenging medical cases. Unfortunately, her intermediate limbic brain judgment was impaired when evaluating Brandon. This is a dopamine effect. We know this from our experience with schizophrenia. When we block dopamine receptors, rational thinking improves.

*Memory*: The neurotransmitter epinephrine significantly enhances the intermediate limbic brain memory. It causes us to remember our first date, our first kiss, our first car and so forth, many decades after the experience.

Thirty-five years later, I remember so vividly all the details of meeting my first love. This is an epinephrine effect on my intermediate limbic brain memory. I also still clearly recall how I met my wife, nearly a quarter of a century ago. I was in a church basement at some function, talking to a friend, when I saw her walking by. My interest piqued, I asked my friend if he knew who the woman was and why I hadn't seen her before.

He said, "Yes, I know her. She always sings in the choir, in the upper balcony, then leaves right after."

I became a choir singer the next week, sitting in the upper balcony and nauseating other choir members with my voice. Undeterred, I asked for lessons. Three months later, we were married! That was a quarter century ago—(Wait a minute. It feels like only a couple of months ago.)

More recently, just recently in fact, I saw the effect of love on memory. A man of past eighty, Roy was sent to see me because of memory problems. Roy could no longer drive, since he'd become unable to find his way back home. He wasn't sure if he had three or four children, but remembered that one of his children was a doctor, just not which one—or what specialty or state in which his son practiced. Not unexpectedly, Roy scored very poorly on a memory test called the "Mini Mental Status Examination."

When I asked him whether he was married, his face immediately brightened and he answered with an emphatic, "Yes, I've been married to Maria for fifty-five years." No memory concerns here: Roy could recall in fine detail the party where they met, what dress Maria was wearing, what hairstyle she had. He recalled what drinks they ordered that night, the song to which they danced.

Without my prompting, Roy began singing to me what he termed his favorite song ever.

*Maria, the most beautiful sound I ever heard*
*Maria, Maria, Maria, Maria*
*All the beautiful sounds of the world in a single word*
*Maria, Maria, Maria, Maria, Maria, Maria, Maria*
*I just met a girl named Maria*
*And suddenly that name will never be the same to me*
*Maria, I just kissed a girl named Maria*
*And suddenly I found how wonderful a sound can be*
*Maria, say it loud and there's music playing*
*Say it soft and it's almost like praying*
*Maria, I'll never stop saying Maria*
*Maria, Maria, Maria*
*Maria the most beautiful sound I ever heard, Maria.*

This fellow, who couldn't recall his own children or the way home, sang that song without one mistake or even the slightest pause. But then perhaps it's understandable. These were all the fine details of his love story and his love song for his beloved mate.

## Other Falling-in-Love Manifestations

In the last chapter, I described the locus ceruleus as an old reptilian brain center that releases norepinephrine.[6] As a quick refresher, norepinephrine causes the loss of sleep associated with love, makes us more attentive to the beloved, makes us feel that we have more energy, and causes the trembling feeling we feel when we first fall in love. The loss of appetite seen in early romance is also caused by the effect of norepinephrine on the hypothalamus. Norepinephrine causes a sudden increase in heart rate and increased sweating, all associated with seeing the beloved.

The effect of excess monoamines (epinephrine, norepinephrine, dopamine, and serotonin) ceases in about two years, when we start to run out of excess monoamines from our brain stores or the brain receptors decrease their response to monoamines. Like the man who's using his savings to buy nice gifts for his beloved woman, eventually all his savings will run out. The time will come when there are no more gifts coming, and he'll revert to his normal income and give few or no more gifts. In a similar way, the monoamine stores are depleted. We usually have enough stored for about two years, and the euphoria, illusions and delusions, and so forth will disappear at that time. The feeling of falling in love ends then.

> *Falling in love is the most wonderful feeling we can ever have. If you are lucky enough to fall in love, then enjoy it to the maximum, while it lasts.*

But please make sure you aren't blinded by the monoamines' effect on your intermediate limbic brain, or you'll either lose your love eventually or live a miserable life with the wrong person.

This isn't modern advice, actually, and the risk of choosing the wrong person has always been present in humanity. Let's go back to the story of Inanna and Dumuzi, to answer our question: Did love change in the past four thousand years?

---

6. Quick reminder: "locus" is location, and "ceruleus" is blue, as in cyanosis.

When I gave excerpts of this book as a lecture, I used to ask people their opinion of Inanna and Dumuzi's story. I usually got two views.

A small group perceived it as evidence for the manipulation of women and evidence of their abuse by society since early times. "This is a story about forced love," said one attendee. "She clearly loved the farmer but was forced and persuaded by her brother to marry the shepherd."

"What abuse!" said another attendee. "This story has nothing to do with love!"

Some went even further by saying, "You're just a male chauvinist to believe that this is a love story."

The other group perceived it differently. They believed it to be a beautiful illustration of the feeling of sexual love or romantic love.

I belong to the second group. I believe this story is about romantic love and has great similarity to how romantic love is perceived by us today. If Inanna loved the farmer, she wouldn't have changed her perception of the shepherd Dumuzi, any more than two friends' entreaties changed Nicole's perception of Brandon. Regardless of what her brother or anyone else said, Inanna would find the shepherd repugnant. When Inanna preferred the farmer, she hadn't yet met the shepherd in person. As an example, picture a girl who dreams about marrying a doctor but when she's grown up, she meets a lawyer and immediately falls in love with the lawyer. Wanting a doctor doesn't mean that she loved the doctor before she ever met him.

Let's look at the change in Inanna's perception of the shepherd.
First, she didn't like him.

*Me and the shepherd shall not marry,*
*In his new garment he shall not drape me,*
*His fine wool shall not cover me.*

Sounds like the end of the discussion, doesn't it? But then, after he assures her of his worthiness and his pedigree, she perceives him differently. To satisfy the new brain, we must feel "impressed" by our mate's abilities, talents, and other attributes. We must feel assured of their love for us before we move to the next phase.

She agrees to see him on a date.

After that, she says this about him:

*I cast my eye over all the people*
*I called Dumuzi to the god-ship of the land,*
*Dumuzi, the beloved of Enlil (highest god of the temple),*
*My mother holds him ever dear,*
*My father exalts him.*

Now, suddenly, instantaneously and effortlessly, something "magical" happened to her that changed how she perceived him as a man.

A dramatic change in her perception of who he is, isn't it? How did this happen? She fell in love with him and immediately released large amounts of monoamines in her intermediate limbic brain. The catecholamines released caused her change in perception (illusions) as we discussed above.

This caused her to feel blissfully happy.

*Last night, as I, the Queen of Heaven, was shining bright, was dancing about,*
*Was uttering a chant at the brightening of the oncoming light,*
*He met me, he met me,*
*The lord Dumuzi met me,*
*The lord put his hand into my hand, Dumuzi embraced me.*

If she were in love with the farmer, would she have changed her perception of the shepherd? She was interested in the farmer based on only the new brain choice but wasn't in love with him; there was no intermediate limbic brain consent.

Just as in pregnancy, where a woman can't get pregnant by two men simultaneously, a person can't fall in love with two people simultaneously.

## SUMMARY

Falling in love, or romance, starts by dreaming about your perfect Person of My Dreams and forming a mental image of what you want in the mate of your dreams. To perfect the image you store in your intermediate limbic brain takes many years and many sources.

One day, somewhere, you meet a person who's close enough to this image. Your brain will suddenly release a large amount of monoamines, and this will instantaneously change your perception of that person. You have fallen in love.

The "falling" doesn't need to happen as rapidly as it happened to Nicole, and often doesn't. Falling in love could be sudden, or it could be gradual. Regardless of speed, the excessive amount of monoamines causes you to feel euphoric, perhaps to hoard every item that belongs to your beloved. Dopamine alters our sensory perceptions. You get the illusion that this is the most perfect person who ever existed. You get delusions that this person is amazing in every aspect, and (dangerously, as you'll see just a bit later) you feel that you'll live forever with this euphoric, happy feeling. You feel that loneliness is gone forever. Total bliss has started, and will last forever. You can feel jealous and suspicious about your lover (from epinephrine effects). You will have perfect, lifelong memory of all the feelings and events related to falling in love (from epinephrine effects).

You will not see reality. Your thinking becomes illogical.

The euphoria parallels physical manifestations of excess dopamine release. You lose sleep thinking about the beloved (from norepinephrine effects). You have more energy and feel unusually attentive (from norepinephrine effects). When you see your beloved, you suddenly release more norepinephrine, which causes your heart to beat faster and stronger, and you sweat and tremble.

About two years later, monoamine release reverts to its baseline, to where it was before. This is the point when we wake up to find out the truth: our beloved isn't as beautiful as we thought, isn't as perfect as we thought. We begin to understand that the old saying, "Love is blind," might well be true. We now perceive things not as we wished they were but as they are in reality. We're now without excess monoamines. We have fallen out of love.

So, is it over? Is falling out of love the end of the relationship? No! It's only that phase two of love, the falling-in-love phase, has ended. We now start the next phase of love: phase three, the "falling out of love" phase. We have much to learn, and much to look forward to in the coming chapters about "what happens next."

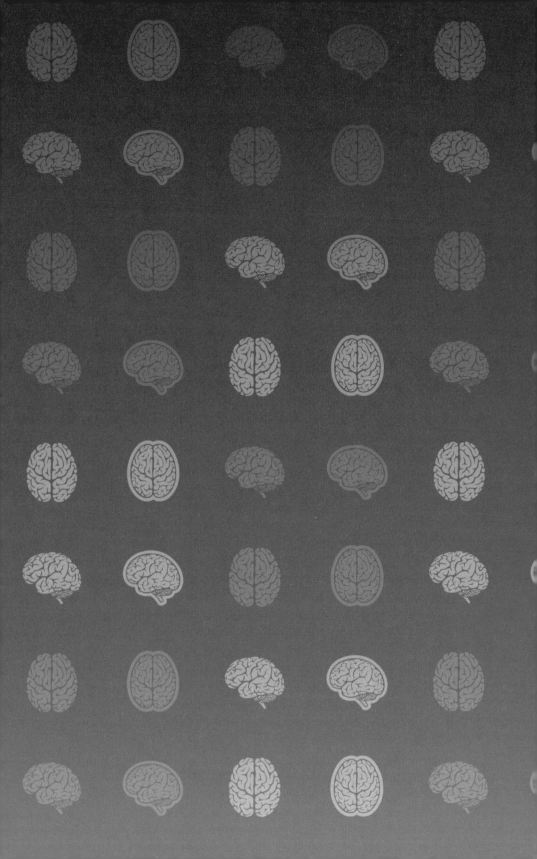

## CHAPTER 8

# PHASE THREE OF LOVE—

# FALLING OUT OF LOVE

In the last half of our final year in our neurology residency at Baylor College of Medicine, I headed to the College's largest conference hall to attend grand rounds, a major presentation about the latest neuroscience discoveries. Grand rounds are presented by a faculty member to all members of the department, followed by counterarguments and discussion by all the other faculties. Having finished my work early at the hospital where I was currently assigned, I made it there early, and I spotted Nicole in the grand hall, already seated. Not having had the chance to speak with her in a while, I went and sat next to her.

"You're early too," I said.

"Yes, I had easy cases today. Haven't seen you in a while. How's life treating you?"

"Overall very well," I replied. "I'm starting to debate with myself whether I want to go into academia or private practice after training … " I noticed the fatigue in her lovely face. "How's life treating *you*, Nicole?"

She saw my concern and glanced away, toward the faraway lectern. "Well … it's not going that well." She sighed. "Okay, I'll say it. You and John were right about Brandon."

Panicking that something had happened to draw Nicole into Brandon's dark past, I said, "What do you mean?"

"You both told me he was wrong for me. I … couldn't see that. I wish I'd listened to both of you then."

"What happened?" I said, not wanting to pry but with the urgent need to know.

"*Absolutely nothing.* I just started to see him under a different light. I eventually figured out that he had no motivation. At all. Not to improve himself. Not to do even the most basic work. He steals because he always takes the easiest way to get what he wants. No desire ever to earn anything himself. Ever! And ... I didn't know how different we are. Not one single thing in common. I was so blind. So ... so *stupid*. I can't stand him at all now. I feel angry when I watch him operate, gaming people, taking things from them, even from his family and friends. I can't imagine ever having children with him. He'd raise them to be like him. That would just kill me."

"So when did you ... start seeing him differently?"

She shrugged. "I guess it happened gradually, over the past two or three months." She turned to me with a weak smile. "It's amazing how blind love can be. It's amazing how I argued with you and John. I didn't realize I was delusional about him when I first met him. I'm surprised at myself. Why couldn't I see that before I ... ?"

It seemed that Nicole had already beaten herself up pretty badly. I said only, "I know. I'm amazed myself at how love alters our brains."

She chuckled. "Yeah. I guess now I'll have a lot more empathy with my patients when they're suffering a delusion like that, huh?"

● ● ●

I also recall this next discussion, or perhaps you might say this monologue, with one attendee at my "The Neurology of Love" lectures.

"Doctor, do you remember this song by Frank Sinatra? Especially the last line ... " The attendee began singing the classic and famous "Strangers in the Night," the very song you saw repeated earlier in this book. As she sang the final lines she kept her eyes firmly on mine, but not for the reason one might think. As a reminder, here are the last lines of the song:

...
*Love was just a glance away, a warm embracing dance away*
*and*
*Ever since that night we've been together*
*Lovers at first sight, in love forever*

She stopped singing and kept the same determined gaze on me as she said, "How can you say that the next phase of love is 'falling out of love'? It clearly states '*lovers at first sight, in love forever.*'"

Her expression turned to triumph, and she gave a final shake of her head. "Sorry, Doctor, but you're very wrong. Love lives forever! There's no falling out of love. If I fall out of love, then I'm with the wrong mate. I should try again to find Mr. Right, and then I'll find the permanent falling-in-love feeling that will last forever!"

There were a few whispers and weak protests from the rest of the group, but I wanted to better understand how she had formed her firm belief. I can't recall what I said, just that it was the type of encouraging, open-ended question a therapist might say.

"Doctor, let me give you another song to prove that once you fall in love, love lasts for a lifetime. I think everyone here will recognize it."

*Every night in my dreams*
*I see you, I feel you*
*That is how I know you go on*
*Far across the distance*
*And spaces between us*
*You have come to show you go on*
*Near, far, wherever you are*
*I believe that the heart does go on*
*Once more you open the door*
*And you're here in my heart*
*And my heart will go on*
*Love can touch us one time*
*And last for a lifetime*
*And never let go till we're one*
*Love was when I loved you*
*One true time I hold you*
*In my life we'll always go on*
*There is some love that will not go away*
*You're here, there's nothing I fear*
*And I know that my heart will go on*
*We'll stay forever this way*
*You are safe in my heart*
*And my heart will go on and on.*

She finished singing and settled farther back in her chair. "There you go, Doctor. They fell in love once, and their love survived distance and time, and even death!"

Little point in attempting to disabuse her of the idea that a song, or a movie, isn't real life—our culture makes that difficult—so I chose another reply, a story about Olivia, a nurse I once worked with.

Olivia looked sad at the hospital one day. In concern I asked her why, and she told me she'd decided to divorce her husband. I was expecting her to next say something like, "He cheated on me," or "He physically abuses me," or something similar. But Olivia said her decision came because she saw the movie *Titanic*.

"I realized that our love has died," she said. "We don't have those exciting feelings we had when we were first in love. I won't live without that feeling anymore. That's it. This is the end of our marriage."

When we discussed other aspects of her marriage, I came to believe that Olivia was destroying a good marriage. Since childhood, Olivia had believed in " … and they lived happily ever after." She strongly believed that love lasts for a lifetime, without ever waning or changing at all. Since that high emotion had started to fade, she believed she'd picked the wrong guy, one who'd failed to keep that feeling persistent in her heart.

It's not my nature to offer advice where it isn't wanted, but while listening, I became increasingly concerned that Olivia was risking her long-term happiness over a wrong assumption. She'd mentioned the story in *Titanic* as her ideal, so I decided to explain to her the reason why the *Titanic* love story lasted for "so long and so far away in distance."

"*Titanic* is a beautiful story, but it is only about two phases of love," I told her. "It isn't a story about True Love, the longest-lasting kind. True Love takes longer to develop than a transatlantic ship trip—that movie's just the story of meeting the Person of My Dreams and falling in love with them. Their love simply stopped at that phase with Jack's death, giving no chance to evolve further.

"In fact, most romance movies, love songs, romantic novels, and the like are about the falling-in-love phase of love. And I agree that phase has plenty of entertainment value—but I don't know of many movies, love stories, and so on that address true, matured love."

Like my group member, Olivia wasn't at first convinced that the "perfect, forever" story she thought of as the ideal love was a story of "aborted love," not a complete love story. Yet how could it be otherwise, with that plot? Rose and Jack didn't live together long enough to go through falling *out* of love so they could make it to that fourth stage, to experience true, lasting love.

The falling-in-love feeling lasted in Rose's mind for decades for one single reason. Yes, only one reason—her beloved Jack died once and for all.

Just imagine what would have happened if he *didn't* die, and they went to Boston together, as they'd planned. Would she eventually discover that Jack's artistic skills might be hard to sell in a Boston that had so many other, perhaps better, artists? Would they start to discover the differences between their upbringings, their different hopes for the future? Begin to chafe under habits about each other that they disliked or even loathed?

These questions are impossible to answer, but one answer is possible: Jack didn't stay alive for either of them to experience falling out of love and then evolve to True Love. The monoamines-induced phase remained forever unchanged in Rose's intermediate limbic brain memory. The same could be said of the movie *The Bridges of Madison County*, which is, in effect, a movie about a severely extended and hampered phase of falling in love, but that made it a quite tragic story. In either case, if these stories had run on longer, each person's monoamines phase would eventually have faded away, as it did in Nicole's case; in *Titanic*, Rose would then perceive Jack under a different light called reality, and the ill-fated Jack might well have been perceived, about two years later, as just another handsome, charming, starving artist with an unknown future.

Let's look at the song again but this time, I'll add notes based on what we know about the brain and love so far.

> *Every night in my dreams*
> *I see you, I feel you* (limbic memory recall)
> *That is how I know you go on*
> *Far across the distance*
> *And spaces between us* (I take my brain with its limbic memory everywhere I go)
> *You have come to show you go on* (Note: ILBMLF stands for: "intermediate limbic brain memory lasts forever.")
> *Near, far, wherever you are*
> *I believe that the heart does go on* (ILBMLF)
> *Once more you open the door*
> *And you're here in my heart* (ILBMLF)
> *And my heart will go on* (ILBMLF)

*Love can touch us one time* (monoamine release)
*And last for a lifetime* (ILBMLF)
*And never let go till we're one* (delusions)
*Love was when I loved you* (monoamine release)
*One true time I hold you* (monoamine release)
*In my life we'll always go on* (ILBMLF)
*There is some love that will not go away* (because you died, I could not fall out of love)
*You're here, there's nothing I fear* (delusions)
*And I know that my heart will go on* (ILBMLF—and forever!)
*We'll stay forever this way* (delusions)
*You are safe in my heart* (ILBMLF)
*And my heart will go on and on* (ILBMLF, and forever more!)

Sorry, romantics, to burst your bubble. This is the reality that we hate to know. You're free to say you don't like this book and go back to reading romance novels and living in your romantic dreams. Of course, your chance at lasting happiness might be better if you keep reading, but the choice is yours.

If you place my admittedly harsh lens on another love story that was made a movie, the aforementioned *The English Patient*, you find a similar situation. Almásy falls in love with Katherine, who dies waiting for him. He carries the memories of falling in love for a lifetime. He commits suicide because he can't live without her (probably from depression caused by the lack of serotonin stimulation from the intermediate limbic brain—sorry, another bubble burst). Again, if they'd both survived and they lived together longer, the outcome could have been different. Almásy and Katherine would have fallen out of love. It's possible that they could still like each other and eventually evolve into True Love, but we can never know. The story ends at the falling-in-love phase due to her death.

We already discussed the fact that there is a massive increase in monoamines effects in the early phase of love, lasting an average of twenty-four months. After that, the effects gradually fade away. This fading away starts the third love phase that is called "falling out of love." This is the period when a person sees one's beloved for who he or she actually is.

This doesn't happen because the other person is bad, although they might be. It doesn't happen because you or the other person is an innocent, or particularly vulnerable to the charms of a con artist. This happens to each and every love. It's guaranteed to happen, unless it's aborted earlier by death or separation as described above, events that can also happen in real life.

But falling out of love seems so cruel, doesn't it? Surely it is the last thing any person who's fallen in love wants to think about.

Why is nature cruel to us? Why does it take away that joyful feeling of falling in love?

Why doesn't the excess monoamines effects phase last forever?

Better to ask, does falling out of love have a purpose?

Nicole's story actually illustrates a benefit from falling out of love, which I'll tell you about later in the book. Without spoiling the story, I'll just say that I'm glad for her sake that the falling-in-love phase *doesn't* last forever.

For now, let's look at two examples to illustrate the falling-out-of-love phase. One is an opera and the other a movie.

## The Opera: *Carmen*

*Carmen* is a French opera. Carmen, a gypsy, likes a soldier, Don José, and throws a flower at him and sings him the Cuban habanera song and dance.

| | |
|---|---|
| *Quand je vous aimerai?* | When will I love you? |
| *Ma foi, je ne sais pas,* | Good Lord, I don't know, |
| *Peut-être jamais, peut-être demain.* | Maybe never, maybe tomorrow. |
| *Mais pas aujourd'hui, c'est certain!* | But not today, that's for sure. |
| *S'il lui convient de refuser.* | If it suits love to refuse |
| *Rien n'y fait, menace ou prière;* | Nothing to be done, threat or prayer. |
| *L'un parle bien, l'autre se tait,* | One talks well, the other is silent; |
| *Et c'est l'autre que je préfère;* | And it's the other that I prefer |
| *Il n'a rien dit mais il me plaît.* | He says nothing but he pleases me. |

Later on, Carmen is arrested for stabbing another girl at her work. Carmen is placed under Don José's custody. She sings him another song. Voila, Don José now falls in love with Carmen. All Don José's senses have changed. He lets her escape, though as a soldier he has to be punished for dereliction of duty and is jailed for one month. When he is released, she dances an exotic dance for him that makes him even more in love with her. When he receives the back-to-duty call, she demands that he prove his love to her by running away with her and her smuggler friends. His superior, Zuniga, enters the scene and starts to attempt to seek her love. Jealousy kicks in. (Jealousy is epinephrine induced.) Don José fights with Zuniga and assaults him. Now Don José has no choice but to defect with Carmen and her outlaw friends into the desert and the hills.

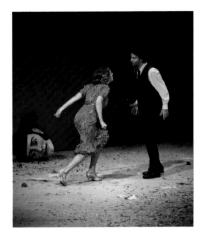

*Carmen & Don José*

As time passes, Carmen falls out of love with Don José, but Don José is still in love with her. She doesn't want to be with him anymore and asks him to leave and go back to his mother. Don José eventually agrees. Since Carmen has fallen out of love, she could make another mate selection and then fall in love again. She falls in love with another man, Escamillo, a bullfighter.

Don José confronts Carmen with a desperate appeal for her love.

| Carmen | *C'est toi!* | It's you! |
| --- | --- | --- |
| Don José | *C'est moi!* | It's me! |
| Carmen | *L'on m'avait avertie que tu n'étais pas loin, que tu devais venir; l'on m'avait même dit de craindre pour ma vie; mais je suis brave! je n'ai pas voulu fuir!* | They came just now to warn me That you were not far away, that you were sure to come; And they told me that my life itself might be in danger; But I am brave! And I shall not run away! |
| Don José | *Je ne menace pas! j'implore ... je supplie!* | I offer you no threat! I beg you, I urge you! |
| | *Notre passé, Carmen, notre passé, je l'oublie! ...* | All that has passed, Carmen, is forgotten! |
| | *Oui, nous allons tous deux* | Yes, we'll begin again |
| | *commencer une autre vie,* | Start our life again together |

|  |  |  |
|---|---|---|
|  | *loin d'ici, sous d'autres cieux!* | Far from here, away under another sky |
| Carmen | *Tu demandes l'impossible!* | What you ask can never happen! |
|  | *Carmen jamais n'a menti!* | Carmen never yet has lied! |
|  | *Son 'me reste inflexible; entre elle et toi … c'est fini!* | Her mind is made up completely, For her and you … it's the end. |
|  | *Jamais je n'ai menti! Entre nous c'est fini!* | To you I've never lied! For us both it's the end. |
| Don José | *Carmen, il est temps encore, O ma Carmen, laisse-moi te sauver, toi que j'adore, et me sauver avec toi!* | Carmen, you have your life before you Oh my Carmen, let me save you, for I love you, Then you will have saved me, too! |
| Carmen | *Non! Je sais bien que c'est l'heure, je sais bien que tu me tueras; mais que je vive ou que je meure, non, non, non, je ne te céderai pas!* | No, for I know it's time now, And I know I'm going to die; but if I live or if you kill me, I'll not give in to you, not I. |
| Don José | *Tu ne m'aimes donc plus ? Tu ne m'aimes donc plus?* | Then you don't love me anymore? Then you don't love me anymore! |
| Carmen | *Non! je ne t'aime plus.* | No, I don't love you anymore. |
| Chorus sings about the bullfight | *Vivat! la course est belle! Sur le sable sanglant le taureau qu'on harcèle s'élance en bondissant … Vivat! bravo! victoire.* | Bravo! What a fight to remember! Dripping blood on the sand the bull they have goaded Returns back to the charge … Viva! Bravo! Victorious! |
|  | As the chorus finishes, Carmen moves toward the bullring. |  |
| Don José | *Où vas-tu?…* | Where are you going? |
| Carmen | *Laisse-moi.* | Let me pass! |
| Don José | *Tu vas le retrouver, dis … tu l'aimes donc?* | You want to go to him! Speak! It's him you love |

| Carmen | *Je l'aime!* | I love him, |
|---|---|---|
| Don José | *Ainsi, le salut de mon 'me* | Then, every hope of salvation |
| | *je l'aurai perdu pour que toi,* | Now I shall have lost, all for you. |
| | *pour que tu t'en ailles, inf'me,* | For you to go running, you |
| | *entre ses bras rire de moi!* | harlot, |
| | *Non, par le sang, tu n'iras pas!* | Into his arms, laughing at me. |
| | *Carmen, c'est moi que tu suivras!* | No, by the saints, you'll not do that, |
| | | Carmen, you're coming with me. |
| Carmen | *Non, non! jamais!* | No! No! Never! |
| Don José | *Eh bien! damnée!* | Well, then! Be damned! |
| | | [He stabs her to death] |
| Don José (rising) | | [To an officer of the guard] |
| | *Vous pouvez m'arrêter …* | You can arrest me away … |
| | *C'est moi qui l'ai tuée!* | I am the one who killed her. |
| | *Ah! Carmen! ma Carmen Adorée!* | Ah! Carmen! My Carmen … |
| | | I love you! |

Carmen fell out of love first. Carmen had a smaller supply of mono-amines to begin with and ran out of them first. Now with normal mono-amines effects, she could fall in love again. Now she sees Don José with a very different perception, her senses back to normal. Don José is just an ordinary soldier.

Don José didn't fall out of love, though. He has a larger supply of monoamines and still has the excess monoamine effects phase going. He can't fall out of love. He can't move on. Don José kills Carmen and indirectly kills himself. All is lost! Dopamine-induced abnormal behavior for Don José induced a tragic ending to falling in love with Carmen.

## The Movie: *Of Human Bondage*

The story goes like this.

Sensitive, clubfooted artist Philip goes to London to study to become a medical doctor. His moodiness and chronic self-doubt make it difficult for him to keep up with his schoolwork.

Philip falls suddenly and passionately in love with a vulgar tearoom waitress, Mildred, even though she's disdainful of his clubfoot and his obvious interest in her. Mildred is manipulative and cruel toward him, but since Philip has already fallen in love with her, he can only see her as the most beautiful and kind woman. Mildred didn't fall in love with Philip, though. Her constant response to his romantic invitations, "I don't mind," is so uninterested it infuriates him, which only causes her to use it more.

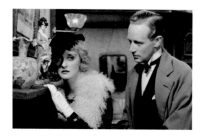

*Bette Davis & Leslie Howard in* Of Human Bondage

Philip's brain, loaded with a massive amount of monoamines, has daydreams about Mildred. Her image appears over an illustration in his medical school anatomy textbook, and a skeleton in the classroom is transformed into Mildred, both illusions caused by dopamine. These illusions, together with intrusive obsessions, cause him to be distracted from his studies, and he fails his medical examinations.

When Philip proposes to her, Mildred declines (she didn't fall in love with him), telling him she'll be marrying the salesman Emil instead. Philip tries to forget Mildred, but his intermediate limbic brain is still loaded with monoamines, and there is no conscious control over the intermediate limbic brain; he can't fall out of love at will.

Philip meets Norah, an attractive and considerate romance writer working under a male pseudonym. Norah falls in love with him, and believes she can slowly cure Philip of his painful obsession with Mildred. Although Norah is definitely a better person and loves Philip, he can't fall in love with her—he hasn't fallen out of love with Mildred yet.

Just when it appears that Philip is starting to feel some happiness, Mildred returns, pregnant and claiming that Emil has abandoned her.

Philip, being still in love with Mildred, provides a flat for her, arranges to take care of her financially, and breaks off his relationship with Norah.

Norah and Philip admit how bondages exist between people. (I call bondage without love *companionate love*, and we'll discuss this later.) Philip is bound to Mildred, since he didn't fall out of love with her. Norah is bound to Philip, whom she's still in love with. (Yes, Norah's brain is still loaded with monoamines.) Mildred is Mildred, not in love with anyone but herself.

Philip intends to marry Mildred after her child is born, but a bored and restless Mildred gives up the baby's care to a nurse. Most likely she genetically lacked monoamines *and* nonapeptides or their receptors, so Mildred couldn't love Philip or even love her own child.

At a dinner party celebrating their engagement, one of Philip's medical student friends, Harry, flirts with Mildred, who reciprocates. Epinephrine still high in Philip's intermediate limbic brain, he becomes jealous. Mildred isn't in love with anybody. (Her brain is probably developed to the hypothalamic sex-drive level only, or perhaps she has genetic defect in her nonapeptide [oxytocin and vasopressin] receptors, a subject we'll discuss next.)

Philip confronts Mildred about her behavior; true to her character, she runs off with Harry for Paris.

Philip again finds some comfort in his studies. Still he hasn't fallen out of love with Mildred; he and Mildred didn't spend enough time together to fall out of love.

Philip meets the tenderhearted Sally. Sally's a better person for him and falls in love with him, but alas, he's *still* in love with Mildred.

(It seems that we have a certain amount of monoamines to consume before we run out of it. Let's say a man has $24,000 to spend on a woman, a thousand dollars every time he sees her. If he sees her every month, he'll run out in twenty-four months. If he sees her only three months per year, the money can last for eight years. If he sees her only two months per year, the money can last for twelve years.)

Once again, Mildred returns with her baby, this time expressing remorse for deserting him. Philip, brain still loaded with monoamines, can't resist rescuing her another time.

Things take a turn for the worse when Mildred moves in, spitefully wrecks his apartment, and burns the securities and bonds an uncle gave him to finance his medical school education. Philip is forced to quit medical school, but an operation corrects his clubfoot. Sally's family takes Philip in, and he takes a job with Sally's father as a window dresser. Sometime later Philip learns that his uncle has died, leaving a small inheritance. Philip is able to return to medical school and become a doctor.

Later, Philip meets up with Mildred, who's now sick with TB, destitute, and working as a prostitute. Mildred's baby has died. Before Philip can visit her again, Mildred dies.

With her death, Philip is finally freed of his serotonin-induced obsession—he's fallen out of love with Mildred and makes plans to marry Sally. Now he can finally fall in love again. Only now, he's likely to stay in love with Sally, fall out of love, and eventually their love could mature to True Love.

Phillip's outcome is a classic example of why falling out of love is as important to finding True Love as falling in love. Falling out of love gives the lover a chance to see reality. Falling out of love gives them a chance to make corrections to their mate-selection errors. If there was truly a mate-selection error, one serious enough to break up the relationship, falling out of love gives lovers a second chance on love, hopefully with better mate selection.

To our brain, and scientifically speaking, it's another chance to find the perfect precoital genes to have the perfect offspring. It's another chance to find happiness with another partner, and eventually, True Love with that partner.

> *The function of falling out of love is to have a second chance on love in case you erred the first time.*

## Falling Out of Love and Divorce

"And they lived happily ever after"
"Lovers at first sight, in love forever"

Writing down these two fallacies about love, it saddens me to see the number of divorces that are based on the wrong belief that the falling-in-love feeling will last forever.

The falling-in-love feeling doesn't last forever. Never did, never will.

This statement is based on scientific evidence as well as on the everyday life experience of most of us.

The believers in the myths, convinced that love will last forever, blame their current partner for the failure to keep the falling-in-love feeling lasting endlessly. They decide to end the relationship or the marriage. Statistically speaking, the peak period for divorces in the United States is at the third year of marriage. This was the period when most people had fallen out of love and had enough time to act and finish the divorce proceedings. They will try again to find their perfect fantasia, to fall in love again, hoping that this time the falling-in-love feeling will last forever.

It won't. Unfortunately, it's impossible to fall in love forever.

If they never figure this out, they fall out of love again and again, blame their current partner, divorce him or her, and keep repeating the cycle. They refuse to accept the fact that falling in love forever isn't possible. They keep blaming their bad luck or their wrong choices.

A friend of mine, Sophia, was married once and then divorced after three years because, as she told me, "We're not in love anymore." Sophia remarried few years later, but again divorced after three years, "Because we're not in love anymore." We talked about it, and I gave her my opinion that "There is no Mr. Right, maybe Mr. Wright." Essentially I shared my thought that there is no falling in love without eventually falling out of love. Sophia absolutely refused to accept this. She believed that if she tried hard enough, she would find the "Mr. Right" whose love would last forever. When pressed, she promised to prove this everlasting love to me.

A decade later, Sophia married for the third time. Four years after learning this, I heard of her third divorce. I emailed her to ask her what happened, and asked, "Will you now agree with me that there is no Mr. Right?" She wouldn't agree with what I always say: "We all marry the wrong person or an incompatible person."

Sophia was now a grandmother and close to early retirement. To my surprise, she emailed back saying that she learned a lot about choosing the correct Mr. Right. The problem now in her mind was "the American man." That American men are all raised the wrong way. In fact, she would now abandon all men in America and seek men from other cultures. The problem to her now was simply the American culture. This time, Sophia would also wait until she was fully retired, so she could devote "full-time effort" to the quest, planning to widen her search extensively and start to look abroad.

She's still sure she'll find that perfect Mr. Right in Europe, Kuala Lumpur, Papua New Guinea, or somewhere else that has no American men! She will be in love forever then. Sadly, Sophia isn't alone. Many members of our society believe that the falling-in-love feeling will last forever. They stubbornly refuse to believe otherwise. Hopefully at least some of them will stumble upon this book, but it's unlikely that even my effort at

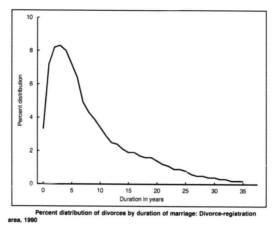

*Divorce graph: USA divorces by duration of marriage, 1990*

science-supported proof of their incorrect thinking will help them see any other way. A shame.

The diagram above[7] shows clearly that the divorce rate peaks at two to three years after the marriage. This is the falling-out of-love period. If three couples decide to divorce on the third-year anniversary of their marriage, the first couple might complete the court proceedings in six months; their marriage duration will be graphed as lasting three and a half years, since the date was compiled from court records of divorce decrees. The second couple could fight in court for three years. The statistics will show them as married for six years but in reality we know that the marriage lasted three years. The third couple could fight in court for ten years. They will show in the statistics as being married for thirteen years. We know their marriage lasted three years, but the divorce decree came after thirteen years of marriage, though the marriage didn't last for thirteen years. It's wrong to claim that their monoamines phase of love lasted for thirteen years, as some nonmedical writers claim.

Please note the dramatic drop in divorce rates after about the fourth year, a falling off that continues as more divorces are finalized.

I wish there was a way to educate the "early divorcers" otherwise, and have them accept the reality that falling in love will always end at a certain point. My efforts with one such person, Sophia, didn't go so well.

7. Source of figure above: US Department of Health and Human Services, Center for Disease Control, National Center for Health Statistics: "Advance Report of Final Divorce Statistics 1989–1990." Please note that "divorce date" is the date the judge signed the divorce decree.

Unfortunately, this change in belief is difficult because our conscious brain has weak control of our intermediate limbic brain. Since childhood, we've programmed our intermediate limbic brain to believe that falling in love will last forever. I don't know, but perhaps if we had started to educate Sophia, when she was a child, that falling in love would have been followed by falling out of love, she might have avoided her three divorces. It might have changed her feeling that the problem is "American men," and not something else?

I don't have the answer. Scientists haven't researched this area of medicine yet, as far as I currently know.

## SUMMARY

We've covered a great deal in this chapter, haven't we? All of it is important to remember as we move forward to the next phase, which takes us much closer to True Love. Since we're covered quite a few topics, here is a quick recap of the main ones. The monoamines phase of falling in love always ends in about two years, though different people have different amounts of excess monoamines and run out of them at different periods. Regardless of when it happens, this loss of excess monoamines starts the third phase of love, the "falling out of love" phase.

Falling out of love allows us to make corrections to our mate selections. That's why we shouldn't reject falling out of love, but should rejoice in its benefits for us and move on. If all is well, we should stay the course, and with time, falling out of love will evolve to the True Love phase of love.

If we were extremely wrong the first time, falling out of love means that we now have a second chance to make a better choice in love. Now we can make another mate selection (phase one), fall in love again (phase two), and fall out of love (phase three). And, if we realize that this time the mate selection we made is the correct one, then we should stay the course, and with more time and some worthwhile effort (and with the help of what you'll learn next), we'll achieve phase four of love: True Love.

## CHAPTER 9

# PHASE FOUR OF LOVE—TRUE LOVE CHEMICALS: NONAPEPTIDES

Unless you're a science buff like I am, you might find "nonapeptides" an odd-sounding name for such an important set of brain chemicals. Put simply, "nona" means *nine*, and "peptides" are chains of *amino acids*.

Amino acids are basic proteins in the body used to build all the proteins in the body. The building unit of a society is one person. The building unit in our body's proteins are the *amino acids*. A set group of people can be thought of as a village. A group of amino acids is a "peptide." Amino acids are the second most common structure in the body, after water.

Just as society is composed of different individuals, there are different amino acids. Just as people have different names, so do amino acids. Amino acids, like people, have two hands: one hand is called an *amine* and the other hand is called a *carboxyl*.

Peptides are lines of amino acids, like a line with multiple individuals holding hands. Nonapeptides are a line of nine "nona" persons, amino acids, holding hands. Each person represents a different amino acid, just as each person has a different name. In a line of nine people holding hands, there will be seven in the middle with both hands occupied and one with a free right hand (an amine) and one with a free left hand (a carboxyl). We can have different lines of a set of nine different people, or a different line by changing one or two persons in the nine-person line.

If we understand the difference and similarity between two important nonapeptides, oxytocin and vasopressin, we might be able to understand the biological basis for the difference in behavior between males and females.

1.  Similarity between oxytocin and vasopressin

    Oxytocin and vasopressin are both nonapeptides, that is to say, built with nine (nona) amino acids. Seven out of nine amino acids are identical, with the same sequence, but "person" (amino acid) number 3 and "person" number 7 in the line of oxytocin are replaced by two other individuals (amino acids) in the line of vasopressin.

    The genes responsible for building oxytocin and vasopressin are located near each other on chromosome 20, separated by a short gap. We separate our words with a space, a comma, and so forth, so we'll know the end of one word and the beginning of the next one. Genes do the same, and separate the codes for different proteins by gaps. The genetic code for oxytocin is a mirror image of vasopressin, so the codes are read in two opposite directions. English is read from left to right, while Hebrew is read from right to left. To someone who viewed passages from the two languages arranged side by side, this could suggest that one came out first, then it copied itself into the other genetic code.

    *Oxytocin and vasopressin share very similar structure and genetic code.*

2.  Difference between oxytocin and vasopressin

    As mentioned above, the nine amino acid members in nonapeptides are the same, with the same members and sequence except for amino acid number 3 and amino acid number 7. This is the only difference between oxytocin and vasopressin.

    Oxytocin, more plentiful in women, has only one type of receptor. This limits the variation in its structure. Vasopressin, in greater amounts in men, has three types of receptors, which causes more variation among individuals for its effect. Could this suggest that men have more variation in their ability to love than women?

Oxytocin and its receptors have a much higher concentration in females than males. The reason is that the cells that make oxytocin in the brain have estrogen receptors on them. With more estrogen release, the number of oxytocin-releasing cells increases, and this causes an increase in the numbers of oxytocin receptors on oxytocin receiving cells. This is like increasing the number of foremen and also increasing the number of workers in each work team. When the number of foremen increases and the number of workers in each team increases, the total work produced will be significantly more. In medicine, we call this *neurotransmitter expression*, which is the number of cells releasing the neurotransmitter multiplied by the number of receptors. Oxytocin expression is also increased by maternal stimulation (love). Does this explain why women raised by more loving parents tend to possess more ability to feel more intense love, with more long-term relationships, than those who came from dysfunctional families?

*More estrogen causes more oxytocin expression.*

Vasopressin and its receptors are more plentiful in males. Vasopressin-making cells have testosterone receptors, so testosterone makes the cells multiply, causing more vasopressin release and more vasopressin effect. Yet, vasopressin expression isn't affected by the man's maternal love. Does this mean that men from loving, caring mothers and those who came from dysfunctional mothers have the same ability to love?

*More testosterone causes more vasopressin expression.*

Could this difference be the reason why women's ability to feel True Love is faster and stronger than men's?

Both oxytocin and vasopressin induce *social recognition*, that is, the ability to recognize friends from foes, and also induce *social memory*, which is to *remember* who is a friend and who is a foe!

The catecholamine norepinephrine is essential to oxytocin functioning. Blocking norepinephrine inhibits social recognition, even when there is sufficient oxytocin. The stimulation (increase) of norepinephrine enhances social recognition. Is the norepinephrine phase seen with falling in love produced for the purpose of enhancing the oxytocin functioning, to more fully enhance the final True Love phase?

Both nonapeptides cause social bonding (monogamy) among pairs. The two systems communicate and change each other. However, oxytocin decreases aggression, while vasopressin increases aggression. This is probably the reason why men are more aggressive than women.

*Oxytocin has more effects on females, while vasopressin has more effects on males. This difference is responsible for many biological differences between male and female behaviors.*

Moving forward, I'd like you to remember that females have a lot of oxytocin and a bit of vasopressin. Males have a lot of vasopressin, but also some oxytocin. From now on, when I say "nonapeptides," I mean "oxytocin in females and vasopressin in males." This is similar to the common use of saying "sex hormone" to refer to estrogen in women and testosterone in men.

## Vasopressin

*Vaso* means blood "vessel." *Pressin* means increases in "pressure" in the vessel. If we give artificial vasopressin to people, it could cause severe water intoxication. This risk resulted in fewer studies done using vasopressin as compared to the much safer oxytocin. Hence, you'll be learning more about oxytocin than vasopressin. Just remember that both chemicals have similar effects.

# Oxytocin

We've strayed a bit into the brain chemicals, but don't think I've forgotten about our main subject. Now let's look at oxytocin in more detail to understand how oxytocin affects love.

## History of Oxytocin and Love: What a Mouse Can Teach Us

When I went to medical school in the 1970s, I was taught about oxytocin. In Greek, *oxys tokos* means "quick birth." I learned that two Nobel Prizes were awarded for oxytocin, one for its discovery, and one for its sequencing and synthesis (how to artificially make it). I was taught that when a mother is in labor, oxytocin is released from the back of the pituitary gland (a part of the intermediate limbic brain) and into the blood (thus, it's called a hormone) in massive amounts, to promote uterine contractions to induce and maintain labor. If a mother's labor stops progressing or labor progress slows, we give her intravenous (IV) oxytocin. It's also responsible for promoting lactation. We know that stimulating the nipples, for example by a baby's sucking, causes oxytocin release and more milk production.

So, while oxytocin has vital, even life-saving functions, I was never taught that oxytocin has anything to do with love. It was up to a mouse to teach me and other researchers of that equally important use.

In the 1990s, animal biologists discovered that one species of field mouse—called a "vole"—is monogamous in one part of the United States, the prairies, but is promiscu-

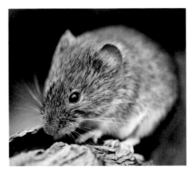

*A vole*

ous in another part of the United States, the mountainous West. The first is called a *prairie vole* and the other the *montane vole*. Scientists knew about voles from previous research on the sleeping sickness disease, since voles' sleep has similarity to human sleep physiology.

The male prairie vole mates with his chosen female prairie vole for twenty-four hours. After that, they bond for their entire lives, which is usually six months to two years. They stay close together, cuddling and grooming each other for hours. If the female prairie vole dies, the male usually doesn't take another female. In contrast, when their montane cousins mate, the male goes his own way, and the female doesn't seem to care. When the montane vole wants to mate again, he takes the next available female vole. Male montane voles don't desire to be with former female mates any more or any less than with any new female vole.

Scientists realized that if we figured out why one group of voles mates for life and seems to love each other while the other group, genetically similar but with very minor gene differences, doesn't mate for life, then we might understand what makes the animals love and bond.

Further scientific studies found that when prairie voles have sex, they release oxytocin in their brains. After that release, the prairie voles become lifelong partners. If we block the oxytocin receptors in their brains, a new pair of prairie voles can mate and release oxytocin but won't bond to each other. They become like the montane voles, one-night-standers, promiscuous, knowing no love or bonding.

Now if we have two prairie voles next to each other that have never mated before and prevent them from mating, but we give them oxytocin injections in the brain, they bond together for life, without ever mating.

Based on these findings, scientists thought that converting promiscuous montane voles into monogamous prairie voles would be simple. If we gave oxytocin injections to the montane voles, they'd mate and bond for

## Voles Comparisons

| Name | Prairie Vole | Montane Vole |
|---|---|---|
| Appearance | | |
| Geographic location | USA Prairies | USA Mountainous West |
| Mating behavior | Monogomous | Promiscuous |
| Oxytocin released | Yes | Yes |
| Oxytocin receptor present | Yes | No |

life! This didn't happen. The montane voles continued to be promiscuous. But why? With further studies, scientists found that the montane voles released oxytocin in the same degree as their cousins the prairie voles did. Subsequent studies of the montane voles' brains found that the montane voles have no *receptors* for oxytocin in their intermediate limbic brain at all, while the prairie voles have *many* oxytocin receptors. Mystery solved. All the oxytocin in the world won't work if there is no receptor to receive it.

## Pair-Bonding

In further studies of promiscuous white-footed mice and promiscuous rhesus monkeys, scientists found that these animals don't have a receptor called *VPR1A* (vasopressin receptors number 1, subtype a) in their sexually dimorphic nucleus, the pair-bonding center in their intermediate limbic brain maestro, the *hypothalamus*. We know from previous discussion of "the vole mystery" that if you release a neurotransmitter but block its receptors, nothing will happen. It's the same as having no vasopressin at all. An analogy is, if you have many keys but all the locks have their keyholes sealed, the keys are useless. No doors will be opened.

However, transplanting the gene codes for these vasopressin receptors into the intermediate limbic brains of montane voles made them mate with one partner only, and they preferred that mate in future mating. For the montane voles at least, promiscuity seems curable.

Genetic studies on prairie voles and humans revealed a variation in this vasopressin genetic code, caused by a variation in pair-bonding ability. We know that different people have different abilities in bonding with another mate. The same mate can't bond with a specific mate better than another mate. Their bonding depends on the amount of genetic codes they have and not on their mate or their mate's genes. You'll read more about this later.

*In conclusion, nonapeptides promote pair-bonding.*

## Monogamy

Monogamy is caused by nonapeptide-receptor binding that induces bonding and identification with only one mate. The binding between nonapeptides and the nonapeptide receptor is very strong and lasts for a long time but isn't permanent. It can eventually weaken if you don't keep adding more nonapeptides to the receptors to replace worn out nonapeptides. Many wise people learned not to date or marry a person who has recently lost his or her mate. They prefer to wait until the separation from the previous mate has lasted long enough, usually two to three years, attributing the desire to wait to allow the potential mate to complete the grieving process. Though unconscious, they want most of the existing nonapeptides to unlatch from these receptors, so they can fill the receptors with their own nonapeptides.

*Nonapeptides promote monogamy.*

## Bonding and Identification

Studies of sheep showed that after parturition (birthing), mothers exhibit the usual and expected love and care for their offspring. Yet, if oxytocin receptor *blockers* are given at the time of delivery, the mother won't have loving and caring behavior toward her offspring. The sheep will act like reptiles, emotionally disinterested and detached from their own offspring.

Scientists did further studies on this. A virgin female sheep normally doesn't exhibit caring behavior toward foreign lambs—ones to which she didn't give birth. However, if oxytocin is injected in the sheep's spinal fluid to reach its intermediate limbic brain, that sheep will care for a foreign lamb given to her as if the lamb is her own.

We now believe that the massive amount of oxytocin released by the overstretching of the birth canal during delivery of a new child and the further release of oxytocin with lactation for a few months afterward causes the very strong bonding and identification of the mother with her child. Strong bonding means that if you offer the mother one billion dollars for the child, she will immediately reject that. The bonding is so powerful, a mother will likely say, "I would rather die than give my child away for anything on earth."

The mother also has an exceedingly strong identification with that one particular child. For example, if you tell a mother who has a child that stutters, that you will exchange her child for an identical child who doesn't stutter in addition to the billion dollars, she will immediately reject the exchange. She uniquely identifies with that one particular child, and no other child, no matter how much better it might be, can ever replace that one particular, unique child of hers. This is a strong identification with one unique child and an unbreakable bond. The same happens with our beloved mate in True Love, bonding intensely to only one person.

*Nonapeptides promote bonding and identification.*

## Trust

We know from experience that paranoid people who don't trust their spouses have difficulty bonding with and loving them. Social bonding requires trust.

A human study was done on people playing of chance. When given oxytocin nasal spray, they trusted other players with their money, even strangers, much more than when not given the oxytocin nasal spray.

*Nonapeptides promote trust.*

## Passion

Studies have proven that oxytocin levels increase in both human sexes at orgasm. Dopamine release during sex causes orgasm, which releases nonapeptides. Thus, orgasm through nonapeptide release promotes monogamy and bonding. Could this be why some people continue to call having sex "making love," an expression that came long before neuroscience discoveries?

Studies prove that skin stimulation by massaging, touching, kissing, hugging, and cuddling causes an increase in oxytocin levels, coming from increased oxytocin release in the intermediate limbic brain, thus causing more bonding and identification.

Studies prove that laughter increases oxytocin release in the person who is laughing. Have you heard of people putting in their personal ads, "Must have a sense of humor"? They meant, "You must help me release lots of nonapeptides so I can love you more!"

*Sex, intimacy, and laughter promote nonapeptide release in the intermediate limbic brain, thus promoting bonding and monogamy.*

## Harmonious Marital Relationship

Studies proved that nonapeptides cause less conflict among couples in a relationship. Thus, nonapeptides cause fewer marital conflicts. It was also proven that nonapeptides enhance communication between couples during marital conflicts.

## Calmness

Oxytocin was found to induce a sense of calm. In a cage full of anxious rats, if one rat is injected with oxytocin, it becomes much calmer than the others. The calm state can even spread to other rats in the cage. Doesn't the mother need calm to deal with a continuously crying baby? Don't we need calm to deal with an upset spouse?

*Nonapeptides promote a harmonious marital relationship and calmness.*

## Changed Perception of Partner

Scientists tested twenty volunteer heterosexual men, each in a monogamous relationship of about three years' duration. They used a computer program to record answers to questions about each image as the men viewed it. Some were given a nasal spray containing oxytocin, and some were given a salt-and-water nasal spray (placebo). No subject knew whether he was receiving oxytocin or the placebo. The study was done twice to confirm the findings.

In the first study, each male was shown a photograph of his female partner, a photograph of an unfamiliar female, and a third photograph of a house. A group of judges selected the unfamiliar female to be of similar attractiveness to the male's own female partner. Each photograph was presented twenty-four times, at random. After each visualization, the researcher asked the volunteer male to rate how attractive each female image was and how erotic he felt about her.

They found that all the males rated their female partners as more attractive and erotic after taking the oxytocin than before. They all rated the similarly attractive yet unfamiliar female as less attractive and less erotic after taking oxytocin.

The researchers repeated that study with three images: the female partner, an unknown, similarly attractive female, and this time, instead of a photograph of a house, the image was of a female acquaintance the men knew. Again, some men randomly received the oxytocin and some men received the placebo. Again, males who inhaled oxytocin perceived their beloved partners as more attractive and erotic than others. Males felt that the other females, whether unknown or known to them, were less attractive and less erotic when they were given oxytocin than when given the placebo. Who wants to downgrade to a less attractive, less erotic partner? Nobody, of course! The men felt that, "My partner is the most beautiful and sexy one on this earth!"

*Oxytocin makes us perceive our loved one as more attractive and more erotic.*

In another study, single men and men in monogamous, loving relations were examined for the distance they kept from attractive women and the amount of time they gazed at them before and after using oxytocin injections. This was done by the physical presence of these women, and later by photographs of the same women. The researchers measured the time the men spent looking at these attractive women and the physical distance kept from these women when talking to them, before and after taking the oxytocin injections. The result: the men in monogamous, loving relationships spent less time looking at these women and stayed farther back when talking to them after the oxytocin injection than before. As expected, single men kept the same distance from these women, and spent the same time looking at them, whether given oxytocin or not. The single men were already at the closest distance allowed by their culture.

*Oxytocin makes a man less interested in other women and causes him to keep a longer distance from them.*

*Dopamine has short-term effects, but nonapeptides have long-term effects on dopamine release.*

We need oxytocin in all phases of our life. We need it to be born. We need it to learn love from our parents. We need it to enjoy playing. We

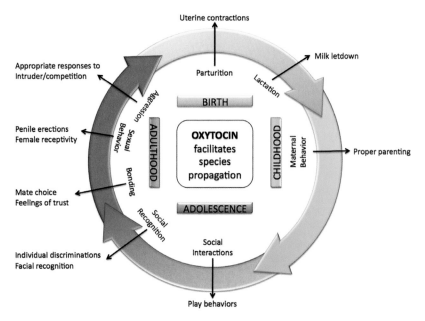

*Oxytocin is needed throughout our life cycle.*

need it to love and reproduce. Its functions change over our life, but we continue to need oxytocin during our entire life cycle.

## SUMMARY

Nonapeptides are chemical substances. As a neurotransmitter in our intermediate limbic brain, they are scientifically proven to be responsible for the everlasting feeling of True Love. Studies of the monogamous prairie vole proved this. Their cousin, the montane vole, is promiscuous because it has no receptors (receivers) for oxytocin, due to the lack of a gene. This was proved in white-footed mice and rhesus monkeys as well. Humans have variations in the amount of these receivers, based on their genes. Nonapeptides are proven to promote pair-bonding, monogamy, parental bonding, and identification with their offspring and a beloved mate. Nonapeptides are proven to promote trust, a harmonious relationship, and calm.

Intimacy and laughter are proven to promote nonapeptide release, causing more of the above. Nonapeptides affect our perception as well, making us feel that our partner is the most beautiful and sexy one around, and making us less interested in other potential partners.

## CHAPTER 10

# PHASE FOUR OF LOVE—TRUE LOVE

Eight years after the last time I saw Nicole, I met her again at the annual American Academy of Neurology meeting and invited her to join me for lunch. When she asked me how my life had been in the past eight years, it was hard to find a quick way to summarize. Finally, I said, "Life's going really well for me. I'm in private practice in Chicago. Busy but enjoyable. I'm married now and have two daughters. How about you?"

"I'm in private practice too, in North Carolina. It's so beautiful there. I got remarried," she gave me a knowing smile, "and very happily this time. Two kids, a son and a daughter."

Her smile opened the subject, so I had to ask, "So, you divorced Brandon."

"Yes, of course. I still can't believe I married him. This time, I did it the right way."

"What is the right way, now?"

She laughed. "Well, I learned from my mistakes. I realized that when you fall in love, you're totally unable to see reality. You never feel that you aren't seeing reality, but you're not."

"So what did you do this time that was different?"

"I asked all my friends and relatives to meet him and tell me what they thought. I was nervous, but I decided I'd listen to them … this time. What I should've done the first time, huh?"

She looked down at the table between us, and I said, "One must never look to the past any more than needed to learn from it. I don't."

She looked up, wearing a grateful smile. "Poor guy. I drove him around the country to spend time with my family, and all my friends. I always thought he was terrific, but it was a relief when all of them told me he was a good match for me."

Our food arrived. As soon as the waiter left, I said, "So, when your family and friends agreed he was good for you, everything was a smooth sail after that?"

"Ha, ha. Of course not. I had to go through the realization, after we got married and lived together, that he has certain habits that I didn't see before. And as it turned out, he felt the same way about some of my habits. I remembered your theory that we all marry a mismatched mate. You were right! That helped avoid my panic."

We shared a chuckle, and I said, "So again, smooth sailing from then on."

She laughed harder. "No, silly. After a few years, I felt like I'd lost the excitement I had at first. I started to see him differently. But you know what? I liked what I saw. I felt that I made a good decision. It took a couple more years before the craziest thing happened—I fell in love with him again. It was a wonderful feeling."

"What you describe is a lot like that song by Celine Dion."

"You mean from that *Titanic* movie?" she said.

"No, another one," I replied. "'Because You Loved Me.' I remember that song when I think of any love that endures for a long time, because it talks about events the other song couldn't—the couple in the *Titanic* movie never had a chance to do more than fall in love. 'Because You Loved Me' is about a couple who've been together long enough to face many hardships between them."

*For all those times you stood by me*
*For all the truth that you made me see*
*For all the joy you brought to my life*
*For all the wrong that you made right*

*For every dream you made come true*
*For all the love I found in you*
*I'll be forever thankful, baby*
*You're the one who held me up, never let me fall*
*You're the one who saw me through it all*

*You were my strength when I was weak*
*You were my voice when I couldn't speak*
*You were my eyes when I couldn't see*
*You saw the best there was in me*

*Lifted me up when I couldn't reach*
*You gave me faith cause you believed*
*I'm everything I am*
*Because you loved me*

*You gave me wings and made me fly*
*You touched my hand I could touch the sky*
*I lost my faith, you gave it back to me*
*You said no star was out of reach*

*You stood by me and I stood tall*
*I had your true love, I had it all*
*I'm grateful for each day you gave me*
*Maybe I don't know that much*
*But I know this much is true*

*I was blessed because I was loved by you*

*You were always there for me*
*The tender wind that carried me*
*A light in the dark shining your love into my life*
*You've been my inspiration*
*Through the lies you were the truth*
*My world is a better place because of you.*

"The words in that song describe True Love," I said. "The couple in that song must've spent a long enough time together to support each other through a crisis, perhaps many of them, to argue and then make up, maybe many times. They've had enough time together where one had to be strong for the other, speak for each other. All of that takes years to happen, not just a few weeks."

Her eyes shining with understanding, Nicole said, "You're absolutely right, Fred. That couple now has True Love. And you know what? I do, too."

• • •

Falling in love is quick, effortless, and unstoppable. It usually peaks at its onset but fades away in about two years. True Love is slow and effortful. True Love starts slowly and gradually grows with time, getting stronger over the years. True Love hardly ever fades away.

True Love starts after you have fallen out of love. At this time, you're able to see the reality of your mate choice. Hopefully now you know that you made an overall good choice in your mate. Hopefully you didn't do the kneejerk response of asking for an end to the relationship just because the falling-in-love feeling disappeared. I hope that by now you have released some nonapeptides to start to bond to your partner. When True Love is evident, having children is a more secure decision.

Another possibility is that you made a terrible mistake in mate choice and need to make corrections. If you're lucky, you didn't have one or two or more children to force you to keep the relationship going for, as they say, the sake of the children.

Chemically, True Love is a slow process of releasing nonapeptides that continues over years. Previous norepinephrine, dopamine, and serotonin release associated with falling in love should dramatically increase the effect of nonapeptide release on the intermediate limbic brain centers responsible for the feeling of love. At the same time, there is a continuous loss of nonapeptides by wear and tear. Hopefully there are more nonapeptides added to replace the loss, and some extra nonapeptides to increase the bonding and identification. Now, with time, you will perceive your mate as the most attractive and sexy one on earth. Nonapeptides also make us less interested in other mates. Nonapeptides will ensure monogamy. Nonapeptides will promote trust. Nonapeptides promote a harmonious relationship. You will never feel threatened by another person interacting with your mate. Nonapeptides will make skin touching, kissing, and caressing more sensuous. Nonapeptides and serotonin will make you calm, relaxed, and happy.

You won't feel this as instantaneously and intensely as you did when you fell in love, but you will discover that the True Love feeling is a much more enjoyable feeling.

This nonapeptide-based True Love has been called by many *commitment love*, *a committed lover*, *cold love*, and *companionate love*. Regarding the last term, I have a different definition for companionate love. I believe it to be love among people who didn't fall in love and just lived together for a long period of time. The typical example is those who married for money but never fell in love with their spouse.

## The Biological Reason for the Development of True Love

We have learned that romance, falling in love, developed with the mono-amines system (dopamine, epinephrine, norepinephrine, and serotonin) to get us to select a good mate and have offspring with the best genes we can find. This system will hold us together for about twenty-four months. Norepinephrine, dopamine, and serotonin also prepare us for a stronger, nonapeptide-based True Love later on.

Even so, humans need another system to preserve the relationship beyond the two years of that monoamines-induced phase of falling in love. A new intermediate limbic brain system has evolved to keep the couple together longer, to raise the newborns until full maturity and independence, which usually takes fifteen to eighteen years or longer.

*The nonapeptide system has evolved in the intermediate limbic brain to keep the pair together by partner attachment for a longer period, to protect the offspring's survival until their full maturity.*

## Is Companionate Love the Same as True Love?

Let's look at the following story to understand my definition of companionate love.

I recently had a patient, Mary, in her early sixties, with amyotrophic lateral sclerosis (known as ALS or Lou Gehrig's disease). Mary was a philosophy professor at one of the top universities in the United States. Her disease now advanced, Mary had just few months to live. She'd gotten so weak that she fell down and broke her leg, and was admitted to the hospital. I was impressed by her wise and intelligent decisions about her care without subjective emotions, but thought it was perhaps Mary's lengthy career that brought her to have a solid, philosophical view on life. Secretly wanting to draw more from her wisdom and calm in the face of so much personal pain and trauma, I decided to visit her at the hospital daily during my lunch hour for a "social visit."

During one visit, Mary was busily looking back at her life, talking about her successes and best moments. I decided to ask her if she'd had any major failures in her life that she regretted.

"Yes," Mary said, her expression suddenly sad. "My deepest regret is that I never experienced true love. I went to college in a small town. I felt so lonely and bored there. There was a boy, Steven, who lived next door. I was never impressed by him, never felt he was my dream man. But I was lonely, so I started to go out with him. I broke up with him many times, but every time, I went back to him, just to have someone going along to movies, a restaurant, things like that.

"Steven was always gracious about taking me back. I decided, *I'll keep the relationship with him going till I finish college, then I'll move away and end the relationship then.* I had my sights set on living in a large city. There, I knew I could find my true love.

"Unfortunately, three months before graduation, I discovered I was pregnant. The best solution seemed to be to marry him. No scandals, no guilt, and no problems from an unplanned pregnancy.

"Steven and I raised six children together, children we both love dearly. And over the years, I developed some kind of love for him. But it's not the love I craved. Not my true love. And I missed the feeling of falling in love. So that's my biggest regret—that I'll die with my soul not fulfilled because I didn't experience true love."

Is Mary's love with Steven the same as for those who fell madly in love, fell totally out of love, then developed long-term True Love? I would say no. I call Mary's love for Steven "companionate love."

*True Love is not companionate love.*

Why do people who fall in love by releasing monoamines (catecholamines and serotonin) respond to nonapeptide release differently from those who didn't fall in love? We already know that norepinephrine and serotonin are needed for nonapeptide release and the partners' social recognition, and other functions.

I presume that the brain manifestations in those who experienced falling in love—with excess monoamine effects—followed by experiencing nonapeptide-based True Love are different from those who didn't fall in love but lived together for decades in companionate love. Why does the brain react differently? In addition to what I said earlier, I suggest the following to explain the difference.

## Cell Memory and Sensitization or Priming Cell Responses

Our body has two types of cells: cells without memory and cells with memory.

### Cells without Memory

Cells making up the heart muscle, the kidneys, and the intestine are examples of cells without memory. Your heart muscle doesn't contract better with more experience. It contracts exactly the same way over many years of life. It doesn't learn. It doesn't remember what it did before. You can never teach your heart muscle anything new.

### Cells with Memory

There are only two systems in the body that have memory: the immune system and the brain. These cells learn from what they experience and change their behavior or response over time.

When the immune system cells learn and remember, we call them "sensitized." When the brain cells learn and remember, we call them "primed." Both are the same thing, but doctors in the two fields of specialty use these two different words.

We'll use the immune system to explain my theory about the difference in brain response to nonapeptide release in those exposed to the monoamines phase of love, and those who didn't fall in love.

To explain the theory, I'll use a disease well known to the public: an allergy to peanuts. A person eats peanuts for a while, then starts to have allergic problems with them. With time, the reaction keeps increasing, and eventually could be massive or even fatal. We all heard the story of a girl who had a peanut allergy. She kissed her boyfriend, who'd eaten a peanut butter sandwich earlier in the day. Her body reacted so massively to the very tiny amount of the peanut butter that she died.

Now what happened medically? When she ate peanuts, her immune cells didn't like it. These cells started to react to the peanuts. Every time she ate peanuts, the immune cells "improved" their reaction. This stronger reaction eventually induced a massive, body-harming immune

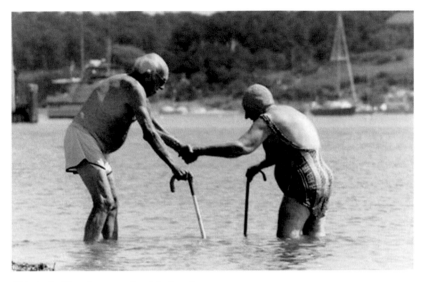

*This is the True Love we should all seek.*

reaction. The immune cells "learned" about the peanuts, remembered the experience, and continued to intensify their reactions. In other words, because of memory in the cells, their reaction changed to a totally different one—in the case of this girl, a lethal one.

I propose that the same happens with brain cells: the brain cells react differently after being sensitized or "primed" by monoamines. When nonapeptide-receiving cells are exposed to excess norepinephrine, dopamine, and serotonin effects, they gradually change their response to nonapeptide release to be more intense, with more intense nonapeptide-induced behaviors. We know that cells that release oxytocin have dopamine receptors on them, which can influence their release of oxytocin. This is one likely explanation for the difference in the reaction of brain cells primed by prior monoamines exposure and those not primed by prior monoamines exposure. It's my opinion that these differences separate True Love from companionate love.[8]

True Love starts with a massive increase in monoamines effects that changes the future response to the nonapeptides release. Falling in love could be a preparatory phase in True Love, because True Love thrives with massive, continuous nonapeptide release on primed cells.

---

8. No research has been done on this topic yet, as far as I know.

*True Love is the final and permanent phase of love.*
*It should last you the rest of your life.*
*So wait for it patiently.*

This is your goal in seeking love. Romantic love is thrilling but short-lived. True Love is slow and calm, but long lasting.

Once, a person who wondered what True Love is asked me to show a photograph that epitomized True Love. I said, "It won't be a photograph of a naked couple lying on a bed ready to make love. That isn't love—it's sex." I suggested a photograph of an elderly couple, perhaps a frail elderly man using his cane with one hand to support his equally frail wife with the other, so they can enjoy a swim together.

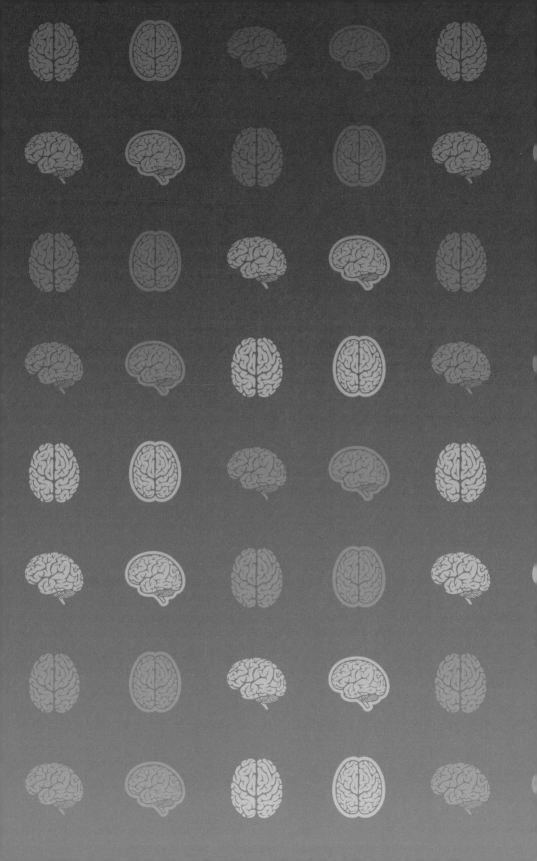

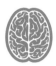

## CHAPTER 11

# WHAT LOVE IS NOT—COMMON MISCONCEPTIONS ABOUT LOVE

Misconceptions about love are many. Some are misconceptions about love among normal, healthy adults, and others are misconceptions about love being a manifestation of psychopathology (disordered behavior). Since I'm not a psychiatrist, I'll only discuss two common conditions of psychopathology masquerading as love, because these are ones I commonly see in my neurology practice.

## Misconceptions about Love among Normal, Healthy People

### Romantic Love Misconception

The most common misconception I hear is the belief that romantic love, which we also call *sexual love, passionate love, hot love,* or just *love,* is the only love we should know, and that falling in love should be for a lifetime. But remember, falling in love is monoamines-based and short lived. True Love is nonapeptide-based and long lasting. Falling in love is instantaneous and effortless. True Love takes time and energy. These two states aren't, and can't be, all one and the same thing.

Many people wrongly think that if we don't feel the falling-in-love feeling forever, then we picked the wrong prince or princess, someone who failed to deliver the dream. Romantic love is the state of our neurotransmitters' illusions and delusions. We can enjoy this phase while it lasts but must know that one day it will end, and we will one day be without romantic love. We shouldn't waste years waiting for romantic love to return. It will never come back. We should instead be prepared to move forward with the next phase of love, falling out of love and then enjoying the wonderful feeling of True Love.

## Falling-Out-of-Love Misconception

Another common misconception is the belief that falling out of love is the end of love, that love ends when the joys and illusions of falling in love disappear. When we fall out of love, it's true that our brain ran out of the extra monoamine stores needed for the romantic love phase, and this loss is permanent. There's no need to feel sad about it, though. There is no need to break up the relationship, either. We just have to work on the next phase of our love: True Love.

## "Childhood Fairy Tales" Love Misconception

When we were children, we were fed multiple fantasy love stories, and of course, being children, we enjoyed them. As children, we lived in dreams, and we tended to believe these fantasies, and no harm came while we were children. The problem for most is that those stories are pleasant, and like most things that make us feel good, we're reluctant to let go of the pleasure they bring, even when those who are older and wiser tell us they're not true, or even when we grow up and have failed at love before, and should know that "happily ever after" isn't real.

Believing that fairy-tale love will happen to us is detrimental, in my opinion, even at a subconscious level. No matter how smart or how rational we might otherwise be, we could spend an entire lifetime waiting for a fantasy to become reality, influenced by those childhood fairy tales to refuse the reality of life and demand the fantasy. Fairy tales make it hard for us to find our fantasia, or to accept that the falling-in-love phase of love isn't permanent.

## "They Lived Happily Ever After" Misconception

Many people believe that love should cause a continuous, unremitting sense of ecstasy and elation and that this feeling should never, ever decrease or cease. Love isn't a continuous sense of happiness and joy, though. True, love *does* have an element of happiness in both the monoamines-based phase and the nonapeptide-based phase, but like all forms of happiness, it can't be maintained continuously, unabated.

I recall an experience I had when I was about five years old. My parents wanted me to grow healthy and strong, and at that time, sulfur-rich spring water was thought to cure many diseases and make people healthier. There are places all over the world that, even today, offer these sulfur-rich spring water spas. Near our home we had such a spring, which poured its water into a large swimming pool. People went there to bathe in it. My good parents felt it was their duty to expose me to this water and told me about a "big, fun swimming pool" we would visit on Sunday. I'd just learned to swim the summer before, so I was excited to go swimming in a great big swimming pool.

When we arrived, I realized that the water smelled awful. (Sulfur is also what gives stools their unique smell.) I thought, *How can my parents ever want me to swim in this filthy pool? There's absolutely no way that I'll swim in this dirty water.* I wanted to go home right away.

They just told me they would leave in one hour, after we finished having a drink by the pool together. I'd just have to hold my nose and wait.

To my great surprise, the smell disappeared before the hour was over. *All the smell must have evaporated away!* I decided. Now the pool was just fun to swim in. I spent the rest of the day there with no complaints at all.

What actually happened was that my brain accommodated to the smell so that it could no longer process the sulfur odor. The scent was there, but its effect had vanished.

This is typical in most of our senses. You go to the sea and enjoy the view. If you live there for a few years, the joy of the view disappears. The same for the view of the mountains, the feeling of a new car, or a new item of clothing. Nothing on earth can make the brain continue to process the same signal without eventually ignoring it. The only exception is the pressure sense at the bottom of the feet. It never disappears. We never stand so long that we eventually don't feel where our feet are.

Aside from that one, no sensation can be perceived unchanged forever, including the feeling of falling in love.

Some people, somehow, have come to believe that the dopamine-induced elation and joy should persist forever. If it ever decreases, they opine, this must be a sign that the love has faded away.

Not realizing or accepting that the joy of love has to fluctuate, we continuously try new things to bring that joy back. Just like the kid at the sulfur pool, if he wants to continue to smell the sulfur again (though I can't imagine why), he'll have to leave the pool for a while and then come back to it again. If the lake view is no longer exciting, then move to the mountains and, after a while, return to the lake, and the feeling of beauty will come back to you again. Again, this will last for a while, but then again and again, you have to keep changing sources of joy.

This loss of joy is less of a problem for those in true nonapeptide-based love. The nonapeptide effect is longer acting, and the loss of the feeling of love takes a lot longer to fade away, sometimes never. Think of your great-grandmother, who was married to your great-grandfather for perhaps sixty years. Their love never faded away. They had so much nonapeptide that it would last them another sixty years, if they lived that long.

*The joy and happiness of love must fluctuate.*

A person unaware that romantic love doesn't last, and shouldn't, might start to panic at sensing its ebbing in preparation for the falling-out-of-love phase. They probably start to think something is wrong with them, or their partner. They want to revive that feeling, even if that means they must try again with someone new; perhaps, they think, a new relationship will bring an everlasting sense of joy, happiness, and elation. Many read all types of self-help books that proclaim "Bring back the magic!" Some people actually end their current relationship and start all over again. Even so, the next time, or more commonly, the next few times, aren't any different.

### "How Much I Love My Mate Depends on Them" Misconception

I once worked with an excellent nurse, Francisca. One day she came to my office with her husband Brian, who owned a phone equipment company. Brian's company was successful, likely due to the fact that he was a calm person who was serious and responsible about life. A previous MRI of his brain was deemed "abnormal," and this was why Francisca brought him to see me. She came with him every visit and was interested and concerned with the details of every step in the diagnostic process.

Testing showed that Brian had a brain tumor. When I told them the diagnosis, Francisca's face turned white, she started sweating all over, and she almost fainted. She cried so hard it made me want to cry, though of course I couldn't; it was my duty to remain calm. She was with him every second of his care. Eventually Brian passed away, and Francisca became deeply depressed. It took her over a year to accept his loss.

A few years later she married another man, Arnold. About ten years after this, she walked into my office with Arnold. A car salesman, Arnold was diametrically different from Brian, being hot-tempered, even screaming at Francisca, in my presence, for minor reasons. He'd been passing out while walking or standing in the car lot. She was as concerned about him, and in the exact way, as she had been about Brian. Testing revealed that Arnold had severe damage to his nerves from excessive alcohol drinking. By the time of the diagnosis, he lost his job. Francisca remained protective of him, working extra hours to support him, and defending him. "He has an addictive personality," she said. "He was addicted to drugs in the past, but he was brave enough to stop. That made him addicted to smoking and drinking, which I believe is much better for him than drugs. He can't help it that he has an addictive personality."

A rare woman, even when Arnold mistreated her, she was just as involved and concerned about him as she had been with Brian. Arnold's health continued to deteriorate, since he couldn't stop drinking or even switch from hard liquor to lighter drinks such as beer, and he eventually died from liver failure. In the same way as with Brian, Francisca became depressed. Again, it took her over a year to fully deal with his loss.

Quietly amazed that Francisca seemed to equally love husbands who were so different, I asked her friends at the hospital, who'd known her during the loss of both husbands, if they felt any difference in her grief between the two. Though many admitted confusion about the similarity of her devotion between the two marriages, her friends felt there was no difference at all in her grieving. A few even asked me, "How could she love a good man who treated her well in the same way she loved an abusive husband?"

Well, I asked them, does her love depend on the man she married, or on her brain's chemical structure?

The answer, I believe, is that her story suggests that her love depended on her and not on the man she married.

We already discussed that prairie voles know love while montane voles do not, and I described the biological reason for this. The montane voles have no oxytocin receptors in their intermediate limbic brain. These montane voles are simply *incapable of loving*.

Later on, you'll learn about the effect of genes on our ability to love. For now, here's what I took away from knowing Francisca and her two very different, but to her, equally beloved husbands:

*Your love for your mate depends mostly on you, not your mate.*

## The "Love Is an Addiction" Misconception

As a physician, I must say no, love isn't an addiction. As mentioned before, *compulsion* is the urge to do something we can't easily resist. An *obsession* is defined as the urge to think about something we can't resist. These aren't addictions, since acute withdrawal from an obsession or compulsion doesn't threaten our life, and an overdose of either doesn't threaten our life. Coffee is an example most of us know. Nobody who stopped drinking coffee ended up at a hospital in intensive care or ended up feeling physically very ill. Drinking too much coffee never put someone in the hospital.

We contrast that with *addictions to substances*. In addictions, acute withdrawal is life-threatening and can cause death. Also, taking large amounts of the substance is fatal. How many famous artists died of cocaine or heroin overdoses? In my career, I've treated many extremely sick people who were suffering from drug withdrawal or drug overdoses, with sad outcomes.

Alcoholism is an addiction. If an alcoholic suddenly stops drinking, they could go through a life-threatening withdrawal. Those with severe alcohol addiction could get, within hours, a condition commonly known as DTs (*delirium tremens*). They endure severe tremors (shaking), agitation, fever, rapid heart rate, profound confusion, delusions, and even wild hallucinations known as *alcoholic hallucinosis*. They could have seizures (convulsions) called alcohol withdrawal seizures. Studies comparing love and addictions found that, in love, there is the release of nonapeptides. In addictions, there is no release of nonapeptides.

Some in nonmedical fields believe that because we desire love so intensely, then love is an addiction. I've spent all my life eating three meals every day. If I don't eat, I feel miserable. If this lasts for a long time, I could even become aggressive to get food. Am I addicted to food now? I really want food so badly, but is this an addiction? If strong desire for food suggests that it's an addiction, then everything enjoyable that we want will be an addiction. Doctors would be advising you, "If it feels good, stop it immediately because it's an addiction." Has your doctor ever told you that?

I don't believe that love is an addiction. I have never seen a case of a patient who was admitted to the hospital for love withdrawal. I never saw a patient who went to the emergency room for a love overdose. Some are seen for depression, and some attempt suicide over a failed love, but this is seen with all sudden losses, such as the loss of a child or a job.

*Love could be a compulsion or an obsession but is definitely not an addiction.*

What I've just described are misconceptions about love in normal people, those not suffering from a mental illness. Now let's switch gears to the other group.

## Misconceptions of Love That are Actually Psychopathology

I've read a book written by Susan Peabody called *Addiction to Love: Overcoming Obsession and Dependency in Relationships*. It's an older book, but no doubt it's one of many similar books published recently. This particular title is excellent, with self-help for people with psychiatric and personality disorders, but love is a normal behavior, not an addiction or dependency. *True Love* is about behavior in mentally healthy people. If you're not certain if you suffer from abnormal behavior, the next section might be of some help to you in answering the question.

### "Controlling Another Person Because of Love" Misconception

Love is *not* abuse of another human being. Some people believe that if somebody loves them, the lover should always do whatever they demand of them. As an example, the woman who demands that her new husband sever all ties with his family, never ever contacting them again, to prove his love to her, claiming she loves him so much she wants him all to herself. If he doesn't submit to her demands, then this is the evidence that he doesn't love her. This has nothing to do with love but is a desire for control to the degree of abusing another person. This is a psychiatric disorder. This has nothing to do with love.

Another example neurologists see frequently is what we call "hysterical neurological disorders." One partner unconsciously fakes a neurological disease to get the affection, attention, and total control of the other partner. Paralysis of both legs, paralysis of one side of the body, the inability to speak, and fake convulsions are a few common examples seen.

The best example I have seen is the following case. A twenty-five-year-old female, Bernadette, married thirty-year-old Ethan. Ethan worked late into the night most days, and traveled a lot. Bernadette suddenly developed paralysis in both her legs, and Ethan had to cancel all his work and all his travel to stay home and take care of her. She assured him that time and bed rest would take care of her symptoms, and refused to see a doctor. Ethan eventually overrode her wishes and carried her to the emergency room. Her examinations and detailed tests showed that the paralysis had no physical cause.

Like all the patients with this condition, Bernadette refused to see a psychiatrist. (If you tell a patient with true paralysis that talking to a psychiatrist might cure them, they always immediately agree to talk to a psychiatrist.) Bernadette threatened to leave the hospital if anybody even mentioned the word "psychological" or "psychiatric" to her or to Ethan, stating she knew herself better than any doctor could.

After assuring her that everything was fine and setting her up to get better by suggesting that physical therapy would surely cure her, she went to physical therapy, quickly recovered, and went home feeling happy. One month later she again developed the same symptoms, and went to the same hospital for the same plan of care, still adamantly refusing any psychiatric care.

On her third admission, by chance I saw Ethan in the hospital cafeteria. He sat with me, and during our conversation he asked me if her symptoms were really to seek his emotional support. I answered him with a yes, glad he had the insight into this; the typical spouse in these cases refuses to acknowledge that there is anything psychiatric in what's wrong. The most interesting part of Bernadette's story? After I explained to Ethan what was going on, Bernadette left and never returned to the hospital.

About four or five years later, I had a patient coming for nerve conduction tests. It was Ethan. Curious, I asked how Bernadette was doing. "Bernadette's fine," he said. "She never had another episode because I cured her."

I hid my surprise, if barely. A patient's husband cures her? How on earth could that happen? So of course I had to ask him.

Ethan told me that he went to high school with Bernadette, but initially liked another classmate, Jennifer. Jennifer liked football players, and he wasn't, so Jennifer rejected him. He finally gave up and started dating Bernadette, and they married after graduation. Jennifer, not surprisingly, married a football player. Just after the last paralysis attack, he and Bernadette heard that Jennifer had divorced the football player. Learning of this, Ethan told Bernadette that if she had another paralysis attack, he would have no choice but to divorce her and marry Jennifer. He told her that he had to keep his career on track, and he couldn't afford the cost and time of repeated hospitalizations. Since that discussion, Bernadette never had another paralysis attack.

The million-dollar question I never found the answer for is this: What will happen to Bernadette when Jennifer gets married again? Will the paralysis attacks return? I wish I could find out, but for most with Bernadette's disorder, the passive form of *dependent personality disorder*, typically continue the same control pattern for a lifetime. This is a type of psychopathology, a method to control another person, extracting emotional satisfaction at the expense of the other person and sometimes destroying the other person in the process. It's not love.

> *Love is a normal human behavior,*
> *not a pathological behavior.*

## Codependency-as-Love Misconception

Love is *not* self-sacrifice. The lover who sacrifices everything to meet the abusive demands of their mate "because I love him/her so much, I must do everything for him/her," suffers from codependency. They look for someone who is dependent, then they encourage their own abuse because this somehow gives them joy. Yes, joy from feeling abused. Again, this has nothing to do with monoamines or nonapeptides. It has to do with a disturbed sense of joy.

Can we find joy from pain and suffering? Yes, we can to a slight degree. Think of the person who goes to a scary movie and who feels so scared they wet their pants or nearly do. They leave the movie hall and tell everybody how scared they were. They find enjoyment in their fear. They'll go back to see the same movie again, to be scared again and risk wetting their pants again. Yes, they'll spend money and time to feel that scared again. Yet their quirk is normal.

Codependents have an extreme form of this fear-induced joy. They unconsciously want to be abused. They can't stop it. When the abusive codependent relationship breaks down, the codependent will seek another person who will abuse them in exactly the same way.

This is not love; this is psychopathology.

Love is a normal human behavior, not a pathological behavior.

Of course, there are many situations when your mate is responsible for the failure of the relationship. The causes are from psychopathology, which again is a disorder or impairment in mental function. I won't get into psychopathology in this book. Many psychologists and psychiatrists who deal with this area of medicine have written good books about these issues, and if you or someone you know is struggling with one of them, I encourage you to read these books—these conditions aren't love but can seriously impede the normal process of achieving True Love.

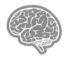

## CHAPTER 12

# HOW TO SUCCEED IN FINDING TRUE LOVE

When I diagnose a patient with a neurological disease, I start a dialogue about what can be done to help the disease, and more importantly, what can't be done. It's imperative to know both so there will be no disappointments later on.

It's the same with love. We have to know what we can change and what we have to accept.

To find True Love, you have to try to manage all four phases, including the three phases leading to True Love.

We will discuss how to manage them, stage by stage.

## Managing Phase One of Love: Finding "the Person of My Dreams"

As described earlier, there are two models for programming the brain to dream of one's fantasia,[9] which is one's idealized, perfect mate: the Western model and the non-Western model.

The Western model for phase one of love, mate selection, is what you've read about in much of this book. The Western model of mate selection is based on freedom of choice and personal engagement.

The non-Western model for phase one of love, mate selection, has existed for centuries in cultures that use arranged marriages as the way to

---

9. Again, *fantasia* in Latin means "mental image" and not fantasy, the meaning commonly used in English language. In *True Love*, it means the person's pre–mate selection ideal image.

select a mate. This method doesn't give freedom of choice. Interestingly, this method has been historically more successful, with far fewer divorces and unhappy marriages than the Western model. Understanding the reason for this success can help the Western model to have better outcomes in love and relationships.

## How to Manage the Western Model of Mate Selection

Do you want to find True Love? Most of us would answer yes! Before you embark on your search for a potential mate, you must do a few things with yourself first.

We've already discussed the development of mate choice when we discussed mate selection earlier, and described it as the unconscious intermediate limbic brain programming. Unfortunately, you can't quickly and easily undo the effect of the fairy tales created in all forms of media, from romance novels to movies. You *can* use your new brain-conscious element to bring reality to your unconscious choice. Remember that you have to satisfy your new brain as well as your intermediate limbic brain when you select a mate.

To succeed in finding the perfect mate for you, you'll need to use two skills: *introspection* and *acceptance*. If you want to find the perfect mate, you have to be a perfect mate yourself. To get there might require some self-improvements. Decide on the things you'll need to change and work on them until you feel your new brain is ready to consider a new potential mate to your newly perfected self!

To repeat, you'll be using or trying to develop two important states to set up for your desired changes: introspection and acceptance. Let's take introspection first, because that's your most important skill to use to get yourself where you achieve that "perfect mate" state.

### Introspection

This is the ability to look at yourself objectively, from the outside, to see what you did right and reinforce that behavior. You should also be able to see what you did wrong, or didn't do as well as you wish, and work on correcting that. This sense is called *insight* in public use; in medicine, we call it *introspection*.

When I was at medical school, our instructors taught us that all medical fields think in exactly the same way, except one. That exception is the field of psychiatry. All nonpsychiatric fields address patient problems in the same specific order. First you want to know which part of the body isn't working correctly. Next you work on finding out what's exactly wrong in that body part. The final phase is to find a solution for the problem in that malfunctioning part, if you can.

This is just like fixing a broken car. First, the mechanic figures out where the problem is: engine, battery, transmission, or brakes, and so on. If the problem is the brakes, for example, then he'll try to find out which component in the brakes isn't working as it should. Last, he replaces the part that doesn't work properly. Now the car is fixed.

Another example: In neurology, I have to first find out the site of the problem. We call this the anatomical diagnosis. If, for example, a patient has weakness in his legs, I first have to determine the location of the problem between the surface of the brain and the leg muscles. Say that I found that the problem is in the spinal cord in the neck. This is the anatomical diagnosis. I'll next try to find out the nature of the problem in the spinal cord in the neck. Say we determined there is compression on the spinal cord from outside the spinal cord, pressing on the spinal cord. We call this the pathological diagnosis. Next, I'll determine the cause of the compression; let's say it's a herniated disk in the neck. Now I have a clinical diagnosis. Finally, I can plan to fix the problem in the spinal cord by removing the disk material from there.

Psychiatrists think in a different sequence. They don't spend time trying to figure out which part isn't working properly. Their first goal is to see if they can open the hood to check the car inside, or not. If they can't open the hood, then it's a waste of time to try to find out what isn't working properly—they won't be able to do anything to fix it. This means that psychiatrists first try to determine whether the patient has introspection. If the patient has introspection, they can proceed to try to find out the problem's location, what problem is causing the symptoms, and then how they're going to fix it. If the patient has no introspection at all, there's no use in trying to help them. The psychiatrist can't open the hood to find the problem, so the psychiatrist can't fix it.

I remember a patient I'll call Mr. Smith, who came to see me because of headaches experienced after a car accident. By way of estimating the amount of brain trauma he received, I asked him, "What happened in the accident?"

"It was another driver's fault," Mr. Smith said. Not really an answer.

I said again, "Yes, but what exactly happened?"

He told me he was at his girlfriend's house until three a.m. It was wintertime in Chicago and had rained during the day, and the temperature dropped below freezing during the night. This caused black ice on the road surfaces. He was going downhill from a side road heading toward a main road. When Mr. Smith stepped on the brakes to stop at the stop sign, his car slid into the main road, and a car traveling on the main road hit him on the driver's side, damaging his car and injuring him.

I couldn't resist asking him, "How could it be the other driver's fault if he was on the main road and you came from a side road and ran a stop sign?"

Mr. Smith immediately said, "What business does that other guy have driving his car at three a.m.?"

I replied by reversing the question. "What business did you have driving your car at three a.m.? Maybe he was visiting his girlfriend too."

He became angry and said, "You must be very stupid not to see that it was the other guy's fault, I'm leaving you right now to find another smarter doctor who can see that it was the other guy's fault who had no business driving a car at three a.m.!"

He got up and strode away.

Mr. Smith had no introspection at all. He couldn't look at himself from the outside and determine, in an objective way, what he did right and what he did wrong. Will he ever change? There is little hope of changing him. It's possible, but quite difficult to get somebody to develop introspection.

Developing this ability is vital, though. Unless you have introspection, you can't nourish a rewarding relationship. Introspection is a continuous process that should last for a lifetime. You can never achieve perfection in a relationship, but you can use introspection to strive for near perfection.

If you use introspection, you have a better chance of succeeding in adjusting your reality—your expectations. If you don't have introspection, there's nothing anyone else can do to help you develop it.

Once you have perfected your introspection, you can use it to make self-improvements. Before you start, however, it's best to do a reality check with yourself.

## Reality Check

While seeking insight through introspection, ask yourself if your fantasia can actually, realistically, exist in real life. If you think so, then ask yourself, "Why on earth would they want to be with me?" If you conclude that this scenario isn't realistic, try to modify the image of your fantasia. Next, make a list of the ten best assets you have. The list can include physical assets if you possess them but should also include those that can't be seen: good character, honesty, solid thinking or oratory (speaking) skills, creativity in some art—the list could be quite long for some of you. In that case, cull down the list to what you believe are the ten most important or strongest attributes. Then, as you know, you aren't perfect. Nobody on earth was ever perfect one hundred percent. So now list the ten worst liabilities you know about yourself. It's unlikely you need examples of these; all of us can come up with at least ten things we wish we could change about ourselves. (Or if not, perhaps the reason why is the topic of another book.)

When you meet someone of interest to you, do the same about your potential mate. What do you think are *their* ten best assets and ten worst liabilities?

Now compare your best ten assets to the ten best assets of your potential mate. Then compare your ten worst liabilities to theirs. If there is balance between the two lists of assets and liabilities, then this is a match likely to succeed. If you succeed in this exercise, you might save yourself a few decades of futile search for the perfect fantasia that either doesn't exist or wouldn't accept you as a mate.

It took years to program your intermediate limbic brain with the image of your fantasia. It will take a long while to modify that image. Persevere in the above until you're certain you've done everything possible to make yourself your ideal future mate's fantasia. Your chance of lifelong love requires that you either change what you don't like about yourself or accept those things you aren't able to modify. (We'll talk about "acceptance" later; it's important, too.) Introspection, then acting upon what you learn about yourself, is a must, not an option. Seek the help of professionals if you need it.

## Self-Improvement

Completely erase all negative feelings from previous relationships. You can't succeed in love if you're unconsciously trying to punish your new potential mate because of negative feelings carried over from previous mates.

Look back at your previous relationships. Ask yourself: "What was good?" Whatever the answer, do more of it. But you must also ask, "What was bad?" so you don't repeat it. Use introspection, explained before, to find out about what you did wrong in previous relationships. Again, if you can't identify these feelings, or if you can but find them too painful to deal with, seek help. Once you can bring yourself to be objective, not emotional, about both the good and the bad, you have a better chance of being strong enough to make it through all the stages of love to achieve True Love. Your relatives, best friends, and confidants can see what you can't see. Ask them for an honest opinion about what you did right, but more importantly, what you did wrong. Don't just ask, but demand a totally honest and objective opinion, with no fear of you being angry or upset. Graciously accept their observations but be honest with yourself as you consider what they say. Be sure to thank them for their answers, and be glad you have friends and family who are willing to be so honest with you.

Learn to be a good listener. If you keep interrupting someone's thoughts to tell a thought of your own, you're not a good listener. Work toward becoming not only an adept listener but also a sympathetic one. The way to do this is to allow the other person to completely finish their thoughts before you voice your own thoughts.

Eliminate stress from your life, whether the source is work, home, personal, family, or financial, or like too many, all of the above! If you feel stressed, nobody will want to be stressed by you. Be relaxed and happy with yourself.

Perfectionism is a problem, since perfectionists rarely find a perfect mate. Perfectionists are always unhappy about their mates and many times about themselves. Be realistic. If you find it difficult to relinquish the perfectionist mindset, it might be time to ask for professional help.

Make time in your life for a potential mate. It takes time to get to know someone, and for them to get to know the real you. Plan to have the time available for both of you. If you feel your schedule is too busy, then you're not ready to find a suitable mate. We always find time to eat, no matter how busy we are, yet too many of us are starved of emotional nourishment. We must find time to devote to relationships.

## Some of My Mate-Selection Ideas

Never settle for someone you never feel impressed by, either by his or her talents, or abilities, or something that makes you feel that they're special for you. It doesn't mean they have to be perfect, but just special in a certain way to you. Spend time with them, and your intermediate limbic brain with the help of the new brain will tell you eventually if this is what's right for you. We call this chemistry because, as I've described and you'll see more about later, this feeling is based on real chemistry in the brain.

Sharing common interests and values is important. We are more attracted to a mate who shares a common background and interests with us. Relationships are likely to fail if there is a big difference in sex drive, athleticism, culture, worldview, money management attitudes, or intelligence. The couple doesn't have to be identical, but compatible. (You can never ever find someone identical to you. That is impossible genetically.)

Gender differences in behaviors and thinking are signs of personality defects. Those can never be changed. Accept that the genders have different brain structures, as we discussed before.

Some of us had good parents and tend to want someone like them. Others had bad parents and want to avoid someone like them. Remember that you are not your parent. You have a different set of genes. Give everyone a nonbiased chance. A good mate for you could be different from the ideal mate for your parents. Don't fix your parents' problems in your own life.

Avoid over-reading people: "Oh my God, he/she coughed twice, they must have TB!" or "He doesn't put sugar in his coffee; he must be diabetic," and so on.

Don't waste time with a bad relationship. If you gave it a fair chance and feel that it won't work out, act on that feeling. Don't stay because it's convenient or familiar.

Now that you made a good mate choice using introspection, are you done yet? No, not yet. Next you have to use the second skill and accept the fact that you chose a mismatching mate. Yes, after all that, he or she is a mismatch for you. And no, that realization doesn't mean that you should automatically leave the relationship. Far from it!

## Acceptance

Developing acceptance is the second critical skill to finding your ideal mate. Acceptance is the assent to reality without attempting to change the reality or resenting it. With acceptance, you endorse and rejoice in the reality even though it is different from yours.

Best that you learn this now, because once you're riding the runaway horse of the falling-in-love phase, you likely won't want to hear anything with the slightest aura of negativity. But it must be said—from this moment, you have to begin thinking ahead to the next phases: falling in love, and inevitably, when you fall out of love.

The following is written to assist you in that preparation for acceptance.

You have to accept that you will marry a *mismatching, "wrong" person.* Yes, every one of us, even those of us married for many years, discovers that we married the wrong person. So why is that, and how can that possibly be a good thing?

No two persons on earth look exactly the same. This is because of the variation in the genes responsible for external features. These genes are only 3 to 4 percent of the genetic code. The codes for the brain occupy about 70 percent of the genetic code. Variation in the latter will be huge, to say the least. As with physical appearances, I believe it's impossible to find two people with exactly the same brain chemistry and structure. Some people take a sedative that keeps them awake for a week; others take an antidepressant that makes them more depressed. This is caused by differences in brain chemistry. We all have hidden problems that are exposed when we become close to another person. We live alone and think we're easy to get along with, or we live with a roommate who's busy with his or her own problems and isn't interested in getting close to us. When a romantic relationship threatens to expose our flaws, we try to protect ourselves by running away from that threat. We want to recreate the fantasy relationship we dreamed about in childhood and blame our partner for failing to meet our dreams of a perfect relationship.

To find happiness, we must accept that whomever we marry is the wrong or mismatched person, and that we need to adapt to the differences. We should recognize that the other person has to do the same to be able to live with us. If you want to find the person who will always feel the same way you do, then get a large mirror and hang it on your wall. When you stand in front of it, you'll find the only person who is tired when you are, energetic when you are, happy when you are, and sad when you are. Unfortunately, there's no other way to find that seamlessly matching individual. Yes, it's reasonable and fine to expect overall similarity in the big picture, but you'll have to accept some differences in the fine details. Not only that, you'll also have to rejoice in the differences, not fight them.

You'll also have to advocate for your partner's separate reality and promote their separate potential. It's foolhardy to think that you will change somebody, even someone you love dearly. You can succeed in only minor features. Most of our personality is genetically determined. We cannot change our genes or the genes of others. Use acceptance to succeed in this change of realization. Accept that no one changes after marriage. Just as you'll expect your mate to respect and accept your "mismatched" state, you will be expected to reciprocate.

### A Special Note for Those in the Non-Western Model of Mate Selection—The Arranged Marriage

No doubt some information in this section might be of interest or useful to those in an arranged marriage, yet there seems a dearth of available research about arranged marriages. So, most of the research (and my experience) in this book is based on the Western model of marriage. My best advice: If you have an arranged marriage and you're happy with it, just enjoy it and consider yourself most fortunate! If you're unhappy, seek the help of your family and community. They have the accumulation of centuries, perhaps thousands of years of experience and resources to help you if you can't have or don't want a divorce, or don't believe a divorce is the solution to your dilemma.

## Managing Phase Two of Love: The Falling in Love

If you're ensconced in this phase, you're probably asking, "What is there to manage?" Understandable, but if you can, please float back down from the clouds for a moment and listen: You can't make yourself fall in love with anybody. But when chemistry connects and you *have* fallen in love, you still need to manage the potential that, at some point, you will realize you picked the wrong mate. When you're in romantic love, you'll feel that you're one thousand percent sure that your mate is just perfect for you, and this is as it should be. But it probably won't remain so.

If you can afford the time, plan not to have children for two to three years. By then you'll be able to see your partner as he or she truly is. Having children during this falling-in-love phase will make you feel wonderful, happy, and satisfied. But you will feel just as wonderful, happy, and satisfied if you wait a couple of years. Remember, if this isn't the correct person for you, you'll be miserable for *staying* in the marriage for the sake of the children. You could get a divorce, but this isn't fair to your children. It's traumatizing to them to have their pillar of support broken down and crumbling. Many children survive and even become stronger people after this trauma, but some children never recover from the loss of their first love, the love for their parents. Remind yourself as often as you can that waiting two or three years will give you time to find out the truth about your mate choice and help you avoid hurting those whom you will irreversibly love forever, your children.

It's unlikely, but if you're not happy during this phase because someone else is telling you that something's wrong with your new beloved, engage the input of third parties you trust. As I've said previously, your relatives and your best friends can see what you can't see. Don't be stubborn and reject their observations. Tell yourself that you're in romantic love and so are unable to see reality.

Enough for now, but while you're enjoying the thrill of your new love, please take time to consider the next section, the one that no one newly in love likes to think about.

## Managing Phase Three of Love: The Falling-Out-of-Love Phase

You should expect to fall out of love, and you will fall out of love. When this happens, it's time to evaluate the reality about your mate. If you feel that, overall, you made a good mate choice, then don't let a lack of joy and excitement in your romantic feelings persuade you to break up the relationship. Don't divorce just in the hope you'll bring the falling-in-love, romantic feeling back to your life. It's not going to be any different next time you fall in love. Look at those who've been divorced as many as eight or ten times. They still, in the end, didn't find everlasting falling-in-love romance.

If things become difficult, remind yourself that if you persevere through this period, you'll experience the everlasting True Love. One

True Love will make you much happier than romance ten times or more. Think of a woman's pain during labor and how joyful the parents are when they hold that baby in their arms. Her perseverance paid off; so will your persistence during the falling-out-of-love phase. Rejoice in the opportunity to nourish your love to the next phase.

If you made a bad mate choice, you'll discover it now. If you don't have children or you feel your children will handle a divorce well, then have the courage needed to change things. Next time be extra careful in selecting a better mate, if you can.

Never go back and recall all the negativity you felt during the past few years. Negative feelings only build walls between couples. Negative feelings are like hate; these feelings never build bridges, but only destroy. Forget and forgive. If you can't, then consider that you might be the one who has a problem.

## Maximizing Phase Four of Love: True Love

To continue to grow True Love and have it last for a lifetime, you need to use intimacy, introspection, courage, cooperation, discipline, trust, and also separateness to get the most from your True Love.

### Intimacy

Physical closeness is the biological goal of love. Our genes are programmed to urge us to do that. We already discussed that we secrete nonapeptides from intimacy. The touch, the hug, the cuddling, the kiss, the handholding, and of course the orgasm all release nonapeptide. This continuous release of nonapeptides helps replace the slow process of loss of aged nonapeptide. The extra nonapeptide will attach to the oxytocin-vasopressin receptor and thus further strengthen the bonding/identification, and so forth. That's why older couples have the strongest bonding and identification, the strongest True Love feeling.

I have seen this clearly over years in my practice. I had an exceptionally intelligent nurse, Lyn, working with me for many years. Our goal was to create the best emotional support possible for patients and their spouses to minimize their suffering from catastrophic neurological diseases. Lyn worked with the neurological patient and their spouse, meeting with them together and individually.

Over the years, Lyn discovered that couples with a strong intimate relationship survive the stress of the spouse's disability better. She used to bet me on her ability to guess if the couple would survive the hard circumstance or would break up after just one or two meetings. Her ability to guess correctly most of the time astounded me.

We consistently found out that older couples survived catastrophic illness affecting one partner much better than younger couples did. Yet, age aside, couples who shared more intimacy seemed to survive the catastrophic illness better than those who didn't share intimacy. Those who didn't share much intimacy ended up divorcing or at least separating.

## Introspection

We discussed this in detail earlier, but introspection applies to this phase as well. In fact, introspection is a continuous process that should last for a lifetime. Without willingness to examine yourself, you can't nourish a loving relationship. You can never achieve perfection in a relationship, but should use introspection to strive for near perfection. Use that same process of self-examination to maximize your True Love experience.

## Courage versus Fear

A good helping of courage is needed when the falling-in-love phase ends and the falling-out-of-love phase seems like it never will. Courage is the antidote to fear and has been for millennia.

Need proof? Let's go back four thousand years, to the story of Inanna and Dumuzi.

Inanna met her brother Utu in the fields. Utu told her that the fields looked beautiful, that the flax (plant used to make white sheets and dresses then) looked lovely, and he could use it to make her a beautiful wedding gown because there was a suitor for her.

Inanna felt scared and tried to convince him that it was so complicated to make the dress. Inanna felt there was so much to do for the wedding. The flax needed to be combed, spun, braided, woven, bleached, and so on. This was too much to do, so they should cancel the wedding and relax. Utu assured her that he would take care of everything and she didn't need to worry.

This suggests the presence of "fear" in her heart (intermediate limbic brain). Does she want to avoid the "emotional pain" in failed love?

We know from our studies of modern psychology that we want to be in control of our emotions all the time. We want to avoid emotional pain. We do it by either changing the circumstances causing our stress or by running away from the stressor. For example, if you're in a bitterly cold room and this stresses you, you either close the window and turn the heat on (change the circumstances) or you go to another, warmer room (run away from the stressor).

I believe Inanna tried to be in control by running away from fear. It's too much work to get married; let's cancel the wedding. She had the fear before she met the suitor, Dumuzi.

Her brother Utu, fortunately, reassured her that he would handle all the logistics of the marriage for her. She need not fear love's commitment; she could proceed and take the risk of loving someone. With her brother's assurance, she felt that it was okay for her to take chances on love.

Inanna exhibited fear over her potential mate, just as you will in the falling-out-of-love phase.

Fear is an intermediate limbic brain emotion. Fear is modulated by epinephrine. Schizophrenics have paranoia, which is excessive fear from excess epinephrine release. Jealousy is seen when falling in love; romance is epinephrine-induced fear behavior.

Fear is seen clearly in humans. Think of the person who gets on stage for the first time to give a presentation. If they aren't confident of their ability, they start to feel fear. I recently watched a movie about a woman who invented a new, self-wringing mop. She had to stand onstage to present it on TV. She experienced stage fright. She couldn't hear people talking to her. She couldn't move one single step. She couldn't see the people near the camera giving her instructions. This fear totally paralyzed the presenter.

Courage is the exact opposite of fear. Courage is actively beating fear. Courage is a new brain function and is a conscious effort. This is unlike fear, which comes from the intermediate limbic brain and is unconscious reaction. Since courage comes from the new brain, courage uses more energy and effort. It's much easier to have fear than to have courage. That's why courage is less common than fear; courage needs intellectual strength and determination. You need courage to be able to take the risk of being loved or rejected. You can never guarantee that you will be successful, but unless you use courage to beat fear, you will never achieve anything in love or otherwise.

My college friend, Lucas, often shares his life and feelings with me and permitted me to share his life story.

When he was young, Lucas was extremely busy studying for college and subsequent graduate degrees. He was always afraid of love, believing that love would distract him from achieving his goals in life. Even so, he suddenly and unexpectedly fell in love in his early college years. Falling in love, romantic love, caused him repeated "intrusive obsessions" about his beloved. He felt the wonderful joy of being in love. But he also felt that these obsessions distracted him from his studies and held him back in his grades, just like Philip in *Of Human Bondage*, the movie we described earlier.

After two years, Lucas, like most people, fell out of love. Being a perfectionist with the perfectionist's mindset, he decided to completely avoid love until he was done with all his studies. When he finished his studies and started to look for love, he couldn't easily find his fantasia. Suddenly, unexpectedly, one day he found love again. Lucas again fell head over heels. Lordetta was perfect for him in every aspect, his perfect fantasia. Unfortunately, a few weeks later, Lordetta simply vanished, moving away with no forwarding address. He couldn't find Lordetta again. Later on he found out that she married someone else. He grieved Lordetta and gave up on romance again.

As he entered his forties, Lucas naturally wanted a family. He loved children. He wanted his own children. He used his new brain only to consciously choose a woman. He mindfully enclosed his intermediate limbic brain in a steel-like grip, so he could protect himself from the pain of the loss of Lordetta's love, and he made a checklist for what he wanted in a woman.

Since he felt that he couldn't fall in love again, he consciously selected the best woman that closely matched his list. When Lucas found "the best available candidate," he rushed and married her in a few weeks. The marriage was a disaster; he soon discovered they had absolutely nothing in common. He's a day person; she is a night person. He loves music, and music gives her headaches. He loves to travel, she hates traveling, and so on. Even physically, they didn't share much. He likes to cuddle; she can't sleep if someone is close to her body. He was a successful person. Everybody respected him, except one. That one was his wife. She believed that everything he did in life was flat-out wrong. Neither one enjoyed having sex with the other. They had sex once a year initially, then ceased for decades.

He was always deeply unhappy. She later on mentioned things like, "All I wanted in life was a wealthy husband who could support me to stay at home, give me children I could enjoy raising, buy me a big house, and allow me to have a dog and a piano in my house."

One day when Lucas unexpectedly stopped at home to get clothes for going to the hospital—for further care because of chest pain—her reaction was, "You better make sure you paid your life insurance premium this month. I don't want to get stuck with the mortgage on this big house." She actually got him to check his bank account online to confirm that the policy was paid up before letting him go to the hospital with his secretary. She didn't go with him to the hospital, since she had other things to do.

When I advised Lucas to divorce her, he always came up with excuses: he couldn't afford to retire with only half his money, the kids would be hurt, and he'd never find love again, so why bother? He could end up without the love of his children, poor, lonely, and miserable. Lucas was unable to summon the courage needed to change things. Lucas never found True Love. His fear, just like the fear-intimidated mop inventor mentioned previously, has basically totally paralyzed him from seeking love. I call him "Lucas El Cobarde," meaning Lucas the coward. Sadly, Lucas agrees with me, but still can do nothing about it.

Lucas's story is about searching for true nonapeptide-based love but not having the courage to take the risk needed. He didn't have the courage to abandon a dead-end relationship.

What about those of us who have already made a mate selection, fell in love, have already fallen out of love, stayed together, and are now looking for the true permanent love or are still trying to enhance their True Love? Do they still need courage?

Of course they do. They want to try new things that they think their lover could enjoy, but they aren't sure. What if she hates it? What if I changed my long black hair to a short red hair? Will he still find me attractive? What if I do this or that? Will she still love me?

You will never be one hundred percent sure, but you have to try. You have to continuously try new things that can potentially enhance the relationship. We need to keep the nonapeptides effect going forever, if we can.

*Without courage, we can't find love.*

Without courage, we can't fall in love, accept falling out of love, and then work hard to enhance the feelings of True Love that cause us happiness for a lifetime!

*Whether we are in the throes of falling in love, or doing the hard, brave work of enduring falling out of love, we need courage to find True Love.*

## Cooperation

You should be able to guide your partner toward a more harmonious relationship. This is a two-way process. Each side works on himself through introspection, and works on the other side through humble guidance. Each side should not be threatened by the other's advice. In the Celine Dion song "Because You Loved Me," the beloved accepted the partner's help and felt that he/she became a better person because of his/her partner's advice and support. The beloved had the introspection and courage to accept the partner's help. Some people are too arrogant to accept help from their partner. They convince themselves that the stubbornness protects their independence and enhances their self-image. They lose so much from their resistance to accept help. We must accept the fact that we all marry the mismatching wrong person, and we all must cooperate with our mate to help both sides—our mates and ourselves—to adapt to the difference.

## Discipline

Discipline is the strength of controlling your behavior. This is a conscious new brain activity. You can't start a loving relationship with one person while responding to flirtations from other potential partners. This is a problem especially in the phase of falling out of love. Commit yourself to one relationship. If you can't, then you're unable to achieve True Love.

This problem eventually disappears as we bind more nonapeptide in our intermediate limbic brains. As we've learned, nonapeptides make us perceive our partner as more attractive and sexy than anybody else on earth. Nonapeptides bond you to one person only.

However, science tells us there are people who are either unable to or incapable of secreting (making) nonapeptides, or more commonly, lack the receptors for nonapeptides. They simply can't make the strong bonding and identification with another individual. These people are like the montane voles—they can secrete nonapeptide but can't bind it to the nonapeptide receptors in the brain. These people are nonmonogamous. Their problem can persist for a lifetime and can't be easily changed. They can try, and try very hard, but they simply can't bind nonapeptides and sooner or later will revert to many short-term relationships, satisfying their hypothalamic-induced sexual desires only.

## Trust

Do you know this song? It was most famously sung by a group called The Drifters long ago, but it's been covered by many artists since then, more recently by Leonard Cohen and Michael Bublé.

*You can dance*
*Every dance with the girl who gives you the eye*
*Let her hold you tight*
*You can smile*
*Every smile for the girl who'd like to treat you right*
*underneath the pale moonlight*
*But don't forget who's taking you home*
*And in whose arms you're gonna be*
*Oh, Darling save the last dance for me*
*Oh I know*
*That the music's fine like sparkling wine*
*Go and have your fun*
*Dance and sing*
*But while we're apart don't give your heart to anyone*
*And don't forget who's taking you home*
*And in whose arms you're gonna be*
*Oh, Darling, save the last dance for me*
*You can dance*
*Go and carry on till the night is gone*
*And it's time to go*
*If she asks*
*If you're all alone, can she take you home*
*You must tell her no*

*And don't forget who's taking you home*
*And in whose arms you're gonna be*
*Oh, Darling, save the last dance for me*
*And don't forget who's taking you home*
*And in whose arms you're gonna be*
*Oh, Darling, save the last dance for me.*

Most definitely, this song is not about jealousy. During the monoamine-dominated falling in love, jealousy is common and normal. However, when you experience true nonapeptide-based love, there is no jealousy.

## Separateness

With True Love in place, the two partners can now live separately at times and feel no anxiety about the potential loss of the other partner. This separateness is actually useful for the relationship. The great poet Khalil Gibran wrote about love and separateness in his book *The Prophet*.

*But let there be spaces in your togetherness.*
*And let the winds of the heavens dance between you.*
*Love one another, but make not a bond of love.*
*Let it rather be a moving sea between the shores of your souls.*
*Fill each other's cup but drink not from one cup.*
*Give one another of your bread but eat not from the same loaf.*
*Sing and dance together and be joyous, but let each one of you be alone,*
*Even as the strings of a lute are alone though they quiver with the same music.*
*Give your hearts, but not into each other's keeping.*
*For only the hand of Life can contain your hearts.*
*And stand together yet not too near together;*
*For the pillars of the temple stand apart,*
*And the oak tree and the cypress grow not in each other's shadow.*

Gibran tells us an important truth: You should rejoice in your partner's difference. You should bless their different interests and give them space to flourish in them. After all, that is True Love.

## SUMMARY

In this chapter, we've given practical tips and guidelines for managing and maximizing each phase of love, from the important selection of a mate, to the thrilling romantic, falling-in-love phase, to the challenging but still important falling out of love, and then to what you'll see as the reward phase for meeting all those challenges: True Love that should last you a lifetime.

During all the phases, use your introspection regularly and frequently. When you're living through the falling-out-of-love phase, have courage to try new things. Don't let fear stop you from trying. Trust yourself. Trust your partner, too. If you feel jealousy, then you haven't yet experienced True Love. Patiently and quietly keep going a while longer. When you achieve True Love, you'll have no jealousy. You'll feel total trust in your mate and of course in yourself. When you feel that your mate is the most attractive, the most perfect and sexiest person for you on earth, then you're experiencing True Love. Now you'll enjoy the most wonderful feeling ever felt.

In an earlier chapter, we discussed the things you can do to enhance the nonapeptide effect and strengthen your True Love. When you start to feel True Love, maximize your benefits by maximizing the passions; maximize the hugs, kisses, cuddling, hand holding, and sex. All will keep the nonapeptide effect and keep the True Love getting stronger. We call it making love, yet it's physically making love "stronger." Keep making it. These things also enhance True Love in the earlier phases of love, of course, so apply them as often as you can, through good times and tough times.

The most important thing is to give it plenty of time. Big or small, dollops of patience go a long way. You can't rush True Love or force True Love to happen sooner. Nonapeptide release is already at its maximum rate of formation. You can't hasten it any further now. Remember that the conscious new brain has less effect here. Just let nature take its course.

*Just sit back, relax, be patient, and enjoy a lifetime of happiness.*

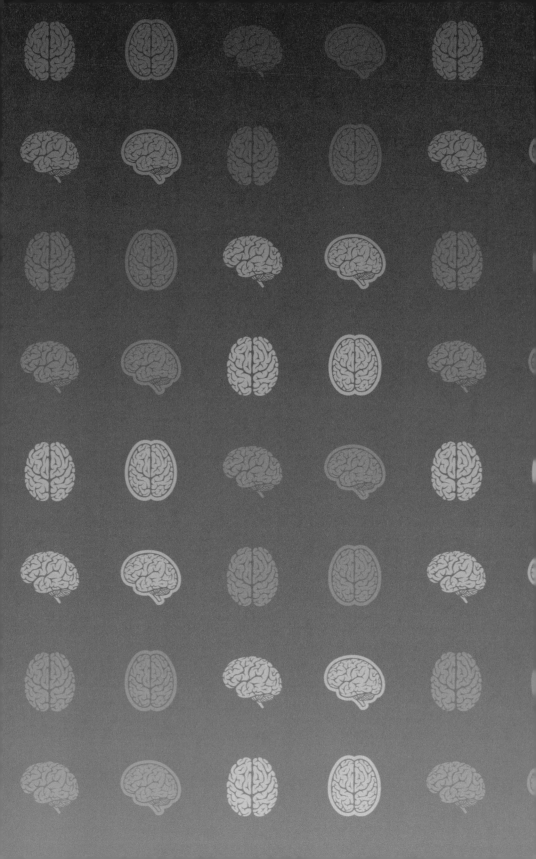

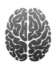

## CHAPTER 13

# THE BRAIN IN LOVE—ANSWERS TO QUESTIONS AUDIENCES OFTEN ASK ME

After giving my lectures about True Love, I usually open a question-and-answer session. Having read this book, you'll probably enjoy knowing the questions I get. (As a well-studied, apt pupil, perhaps you'll even take a stab at giving your own answers to some of them!) These are the most common questions asked.

**Q- How do you know if someone loves you or not?**

I usually turn the question around and ask how the audience members would answer. The most common answer is, "It's in their kiss." The next most-common answer is, essentially, "It's in their gifts." (Meaning, if he or she loves you, they'll buy you expensive gifts.) Some in the audience reply that it's in the passion the person shows in making love. Some even believe that it's from him or her repeatedly saying, "I love you."

Each time, I disagree with all these answers. None of them proves love. Anybody can tell the opposite sex that they love them, can spend the money to buy gifts, or kiss and even have sex with someone they don't love.

In my opinion, the way to know if love is genuine is from the way that person perceives you.

An example: Two mothers watch their kids play a game, and suddenly the kids start a fight. If you asked each mother, "Whose fault was the fight?" chances are, each mother would say it was the other mother's kid. "My child didn't do anything wrong; it was this evil other child's fault." Neither mother is lying. Neither mother is faking an answer. Both mothers truly believe that it was the other mother's child. Why is that? It's because each mother loves her child, so she can't perceive what they do wrong. Everything they do is right. She is a "biased observer."

We've all experienced biased observations. Think about the "rare" car someone bought recently. Now suddenly, that person notices hundreds of cars everywhere that are exactly like his car, which he never noticed before. Another example is the woman who gets pregnant. She suddenly perceives that there's an epidemic of pregnancies. She now believes that the number of pregnant women has suddenly gone up dramatically. She became a biased observer, who now notices every pregnant woman when she didn't notice them so much before.

It's the same with love. Someone who loves you will see you as being perfect in every way, all the time. Your opinions are definitely the correct ones all the time. It's never your fault when something goes wrong. If you get fired from work because you didn't show up to work more than 50 percent of the time, your biased lover will believe it was your boss's fault. He just didn't like you, they'll insist, and that is all the truth to your firing.

Just watching the biased behavior of your mate toward you will tell you how much they truly love you. If everything about you is perceived as just perfect, if they believe you can do no wrongs, then you should know that they love you sincerely.

*To know if the one you love really loves you, no gifts, words of love, kisses, or sex can be as reliable as their biased observations of you.*

## Q- Can we do diagnostic tests for love?

My office employees used to dread me giving the lecture about love. One day I asked them, "Why is that?" They told me that after each presentation and for the next few weeks, they'd spend too much time explaining to people that "Dr. Nour" can't order tests on their mates to prove or disprove their love.

Yet, why *can't* modern medicine do tests to help people find out about their love?

That's because what we've seen and read about fMRI images of love aren't real science, in my opinion. I'll be delving into this a bit later in an appendix, but for now I'll just give a short summary of the problem: These machines create positive results (images) in over 70 percent of cases when the subject is doing absolutely nothing mentally. Literally nothing. Using this technology, they've generated impressive-looking images in salmon brains, images that suggest that the salmon can process human emotions. However, there was one problem—the uncooperative salmon was dead! The researcher had bought it earlier in the day from a fish market.

Again, you'll see more about this problem (including more about the "dead salmon images") later on when I give a detailed background of this problem. In reality, we don't have really reliable tests to show evidence of love in living people. To have any hope of testing for love, we need a more advanced technology to see the actual chemicals in the brain and measure them with consistent, individual results.

The most common brain disease is probably depression. Even today, we still can't image the serotonin, norepinephrine, or other chemicals responsible for the disease. The day we succeed in this will be a historic day, because it will change the way we diagnose and treat this common malady. It's not hyperbole to say this would be the beginning of a new era in medicine. Progress is being made toward that new era, however. We're now able to see, for the first time, a dopamine protein that is used for dopamine to travel back into the brain cell. (The test is called a DaT scan: Da=dopamine, T=transporter.) This test is commercially available now.

I believe it's only a matter of time before we see more of these chemicals, including those responsible for love, in living brains.

Another challenge to developing a "love test" is similar to one experienced by computer researchers. If you want to diagnose a computer software problem, the computer must be on. If you wait until it's turned off, you'll never be able to observe the problem, which is vital to finding and fixing the problem. It's the same with the brain; you have to be living and well to find out what's wrong with many dynamic "software" brain disorders. This hurdle will be gotten over in time, I'm certain. But not today. We can't use questionable, imperfect technology to recommend reliable solutions. Remember that the first rule in the Hippocratic Oath is still "Do no harm." Until procedures and technology become reliable, reporting inaccurate results does widespread harm.

## Q- Can we give medications to improve love?

Put another way, why don't neurologists use medications to change or enhance the way we feel when in love?

It's extremely difficult to enter chemicals directly into the brain. The brain has the so-called "blood-brain barrier," or BBB for short. This barrier controls what the brain needs and then allows only the needed chemicals to enter the brain through the BBB.

We *can* give dopamine-enhancing medications, but we can't make them go to the intermediate limbic-brain centers responsible for the feeling of falling in love. So giving dopamine-enhancing medications probably has no effect on the falling-in-love feeling. We have four chemicals involved, so we need to change all of them, but we cannot. All the monoamines have to come naturally, from within the intermediate limbic brain itself. We're not able, at this time, to reliably change the inside of the intermediate limbic brain.

The same situation exists with nonapeptides. We can give oxytocin that goes via the blood to the uterus and make it contract, and it goes to other organs too, to cause certain effects. Unfortunately, only a very small fraction of this oxytocin can cross the BBB to get to the central oxytocin receptors and cells responsible for the feeling of True Love. Giving extra oxytocin for long periods of time can cause many side effects too, because the oxytocin in blood affects other parts of the body, with only a mild central oxytocin effect in the brain. This oxytocin harms the heart and the circulation. Vasopressin causes severe water intoxication, and so on. Low vasopressin levels cause a disease called *diabetes insipidus.* This is of little practical clinical significance to be used in people yet. Besides, there are many natural methods of doing this, as mentioned before, and as most natural things can be, those would be safer.

We need to find a new trick to succeed in increasing central nonapeptides with no side effects. It's only a matter of time before we succeed in doing so.

Until then, please don't try to Google me and come to see me for any tests or drugs for love. The only answer I can give is, "Maybe someday."

## Q- What is the difference between heterosexual love and homosexual love?

Part of the answer to this question can be gleaned from previous sections of this book, so I'll make quick returns to them here.

## Phase One of Love: Mate Selection

When we discussed the sex drive, we discussed sex-orientation development, how the nuclei in the hypothalamus (part of the intermediate limbic brain) responsible for sexual orientation—the sexually dimorphic nucleus—is present in only one area in the hypothalamus, and that in all mammals studied, this area is at least twice as big in males as in females. This increase is caused by testosterone's effect on it and is responsible for inducing the male appetite for sex acts. Increasing dopamine here causes an increase in sex drive.

The sexually dimorphic nucleus is also involved in sex partner preference; the aromatase enzyme present in the sexually dimorphic nucleus was found to be twice as high in heterosexual as homosexual rams. Also, damaging the sexually dimorphic nucleus in male heterosexual ferrets transformed them into homosexual ferrets.

However, what is considered as fact in animals doesn't always transfer over to humans. Indeed, human studies have showed conflicting findings. We're still researching this area for an answer, and the only difference we've found between a homosexual and heterosexual person was in the sex of the chosen mate.

## Phase Two of Love: Falling in Love / Romantic Love

Studies comparing falling in love in heterosexual couples and homosexual couples showed no differences at all. The same monoamines changes in the same locations in the brain are seen in both groups.

## Phase Three of Love: Falling Out of Love

Studies comparing the falling-out-of-love phase in heterosexual couples and homosexual couples showed no differences at all. There is the same loss of the former monoamine-effects in falling out of love in both groups.

## Phase Four of Love: True Love

Studies comparing True Love in heterosexual couples and homosexual couples showed no differences at all; nonapeptide studies also showed the same patterns in both heterosexuals and homosexuals in the same locations.

So, studies comparing love in heterosexual couples and homosexual couples showed no differences at all, except for the sex of the mate chosen, with the slight possibility that, someday, a chemical linkage might either be found or disproved for good.

### Q- Can we train our brain to release more monoamines or nonapeptide?

The answer is simply no. It all has to come naturally. As they say, you can't buy love. You can't make yourself love someone, either, or make someone artificially love you.

### Q- What is the relationship between genes and love?

*Genes have a significant effect on our emotions.* We already discussed how the prairie voles and montane voles were discovered to be monogamous in one group and promiscuous in another group, based on the difference in the gene codes.

Many genes are currently under study. I'll first make a list of fifteen of those genes, with their medical abbreviation in parentheses, just to show you the extent of the genes that affect our love behavior. I'll then select a few from the list to discuss further; you'll see those discussions after the list.

**Genes studied for their effects on love-behavior variation include:**

Oxytocin receptor gene (OXTR)
Oxytocin neurophysin I (NPI)
Oxytocinase & vasopressinase-processing enzyme genes (LNPEP)
Oxytocin system ADP-ribozymes cyclase (CD38)
Arginine vasopressin 1 receptor A (AVPR1a) (which I referred to as vasopressin)
Arginine vasopressin 1 receptor B (AVPR1b)
Arginine vasopressin neurophysin II (NPII)

Serotonin 1A gene (5-HT1A)
Serotonin transporter promoter receptor gene (5-HTTLPR)
Serotonin transporter gene (5-HTT)
Dopamine receptor D2 gene (DRD2)
Dopamine receptor D4 gene (DRD4)
Dopamine active transporter gene (DaT)
Catechol-O-methyl transferase gene (COMT)
Major histocompatibility complex allele variation

Now let's discuss *a few* of these genes. (I could address more, but that could get quite complicated.)

## Oxytocin Receptor Genes Variation

Studies have been done on gene variations in oxytocin receptor genes (testing five allele variations). An allele is a location in the genetic code. For example, my kitchen has marble tiles. These tiles come in four different but similar patterns or designs. Each design can be called a pattern with slight variation from the other three patterns. In genetic coding, we call each tile an allele. One allele is a certain sequence of amino acids or arrangement of the people standing in the line, as mentioned before. Another allele is the same amino acids in a different sequence, such as rearranging where some people stand in the line. Genes are used to manufacture oxytocin receptors. Genetic studies proved that the larger the number of healthy receptors, the more empathetic the communication with the partner. Empathetic behaviors studies included support-giving interactions such as: maintaining focus on partner, acknowledging pattern distress, and verbal and nonverbal empathy. Other studies looked at the effect of these gene variations on the size of the intermediate limbic brain centers. Larger intermediate limbic brain centers are associated with stronger emotions.

Those with better genes had a bigger intermediate limbic brain center and a stronger sense of True Love. Those with bad genes had smaller intermediate limbic brain centers and a weaker sense of True Love. If your mate can't feel the intense emotions you have, they probably have fewer nonapeptide receptors. Just as in marrying a short person, arguing and demanding that they become tall will only frustrate the two sides. You just have to accept that your mate is short (or short of nonapeptides) and go on with other aspects of the relationship.

## Oxytocin System ADP-Ribozymes Cyclase (CD38)

You've learned about the importance of oxytocin in love. The gene CD38 affects oxytocin secretions. A certain allele[10] is associated with better-expressed gratitude between members of a romantic relationship and higher relationship satisfaction. Another allele in the mate was associated with less appreciation of gratitude exhibited by the partner. Just remember, nobody can ever change their genes.

## Vasopressin Receptor 1A Genes Variation

The genes for this receptor have "code repeats" in a certain area. If the code is repeated twice, you produce twice as much vasopressin. If the repetitions are more frequent, you have even more vasopressin. It's been proven that humans with more repetitions have more bonding with their mate than those with fewer repetitions.

Repeat variations in the vasopressin promoter-region are associated with altruism, music, and dance. More repetitions caused greater altruism and music appreciation, and the gift of dance, as well as True Love.

There are two regulatory regions in the genes, called the *cis* and *motif*, that regulate the transcription (*execution*) of the genetic codes. An example: the repeats are part of the car blueprint design; the execution is part of the assembly line. *Cis-regulatory elements* enhance the transcription of the genes, while the *motif-regulatory elements* suppress the transcription. Since vasopressin is expressed in males more than females, it's thought that male aggression and response to stress is regulated by the amount of vasopressin in the intermediate limbic brain. Studies of humans and chimpanzees proved that more Cis and fewer motif sequences (resulting in more vasopressin expression) are associated with stronger bonding with mates and vice versa.

## Serotonin (5-HT1A) Receptors Gene

Serotonin receptor (5-HT1A) gene variations were studied for their effect on the chances of young adults falling in love. There are two variations of this gene, CC and CG. (To explain the Cs and Gs: the second amino acid in one is **cytocine** and in the other is Guanine.) Those who carry the gene

---

10. rs6449182 in the lover and rs3796863 in the mate.

variant with CC fall in love more easily than those who carry the CG variant. The CG variant was associated with personality that is more neurotic, with more depressions and pessimism. It's all in the genetic code.

## Serotonin Transporter Promoter Receptor Regions (5-HTTLPR)

Studies of serotonin transporter promoter regions (5-HTTLPR) found two variants: *ll* and *ss*.[11] One variant has a long arm (l/l for "long long") and the other has a short arm (s/s). Those carrying the long-arm variant had better romantic relationship satisfaction than those with the short variant. Those with short-arm variant of the gene showed more social interaction anxiety. Maybe your mate has the s/s variant and can't help it.

## Major Histocompatibility Complex (MHC)

Major histocompatibility complex is an area in the genetic codes for cell surface markers that the immune system uses to identify "self" (your own body) from "foreign" (such as bacteria, viruses, and so on). In the First Gulf War, we had an initial problem where US fighter planes kept attacking US tanks. It turned out to be caused by the failure of US fighter planes to identify US tanks. There was a code on the tops of US tanks that should have been detected by US fighter planes. However, sand covered the top of the tanks, which caused a failure in identifying "self" (US tanks), from "foreign" (Iraqi tanks). To fight infections and other invaders into our bodies, we must identify self-versus-foreign cells. MHC basically writes codes for making "labels" on cell surfaces so the immune system won't attack our own cells. If one country has one type of defense weapons, such as tanks, and another country has tanks *and* airplanes, we expect the country with two sets of weapons to be more successful in defending itself. The greater the variety of weapons, the better the defense will be. If two countries want to combine their armies, the best choice is to have one country that has tanks and airplanes merge with a country that has a navy and nuclear weapons. Tanks, airplanes, ships, and other military elements are called *types* of weapons. In the immune system, we call each type of weapon an *allele*. The more allele variations, the better the immune system and the fewer diseases we have.

---

11. For those who love details, the gene is called SLC6A4.

In a study of sexual satisfaction and unfaithfulness in romantic couples, men and women rated their satisfaction with their romantic mate as well as their extra-relationship sexual encounters. They took tissue samples from the couples, examined the MHC alleles they had, and correlated the variations with the mates' reports.

The result was that mates who had great similarity in their MHC had less satisfaction in the relationship and more extra-relationship sex. In the women, extra-relationship affairs peaked during ovulation, and they had more orgasms with men of different MHC alleles than those with similar MHC alleles.

Surprising or not, mates find potential mates with different MHC alleles more attractive than those whose alleles are similar, because a mate with similar MHC alleles will produce less healthy offspring.

Now you have some evidence that you shouldn't seek someone who's exactly like you, but someone who is different. If you don't feel that "chemistry" between you and a certain mate, maybe you've discerned, by scent, that your bodies will produce unhealthy babies.

How do mates smell a good match?

In one study, women were given T-shirts that had been worn by men for two days, and were instructed to sniff and select the ones with a scent they liked and those with a scent they disliked. Man A's shirt could be disliked by Woman A but loved by Woman B. When they took tissue samples from the mouths of all the subjects, they found out that Man A and Woman A had very similar MHC, while Woman B had a different MHC.

You probably recall my story about the woman I liked, but I felt she smelled bad, when my friend, who knew her for years, didn't smell anything bad? Likely, her MHC was too similar to mine!

More interesting, hormone levels seem to enhance that "scent appeal." When the women in the study were ovulating, they liked the smell of men with alleles different from them more than those with similar alleles. When the women were taking hormonal oral contraceptives, they couldn't tell the difference between Man A and Man B. Could oral contraceptives interfere in our mate selection? I don't know the answer.

*The bottom line? Ovulating women can smell a good (matching) man from far away.*

## Q- What about love, serotonin, sex, depression, and antidepressants?

Since we discussed serotonin and love in an earlier chapter, I'll limit my answer here to the effects of depression and antidepressants on sex.

The sex drive comes from the effect of dopamine release on the sexually dimorphic nucleus. Serotonin enhances dopamine release. A normal person with normal amounts of serotonin has a healthy sex drive. If that person gets depressed, the decrease in serotonin causes less dopamine release at the sexually dimorphic nucleus and thus a lower sex drive. Antidepressants, by increasing serotonin, should eventually return the sex drive to normal. I say "eventually," because early in the treatment, we might see a decrease in the sex drive. This is like putting out a forest fire. Early on, when the fireman sprays water on the fire, the fire continues to spread. Yet it's inaccurate to say that water increases forest fires. Similarly, the decrease in sex drive is from the depression itself, in spite of the antidepressants and not because of them.

Orgasm is caused by dopamine release. Let's use an analogy here. The gun has a trigger. You have to move the trigger a certain distance, say half an inch, to reach a point called the firing point. At this point, the gun will fire. In orgasm, the sexual activity gradually moves the trigger back until it hits the firing point, and voila, an orgasm happens. Serotonin and antidepressants move the "gun firing point" backward. Now you have to push the trigger back further, let's say three-quarters of an inch, but it would be wrong to say that this prevents the gun from firing. The antidepressant effect makes it take longer to reach an orgasm but doesn't prevent it. Oxytocin is involved too. More oxytocin causes an earlier orgasm, and vice versa. When you are in True Love, orgasms will be easier.

I don't believe the nonmedical authors when they say such things as:

"Drugs that boost serotonin system in the brain tend to suppress dopamine circuits—the circuits associated with feelings of intense romantic love."

Or things like:

"SSRIs blunt emotions."

"Seventy-five percent of patients needlessly take SSRIs."

"SSRIs and Cymbalta interfere with desire and orgasm in 73% of people taking them."

*Or* that "Serotonin levels in the blood increase during romantic love."

Drawing from an example I gave earlier in the book, remember that serotonin in blood and the brain have the same relationship as the relationship between people walking on Fifth Avenue and people attending *The Oprah Show* in Chicago. Both places have people, but the presence of more people in one place has no relationship to the number of people in the other place. I ignore these authors' listings of depressed people who lost interest in sex when they became depressed and their ridiculous statements along the lines of, "Antidepressants may impair women's ability to select a suitable mate as without orgasm, a woman cannot tell who is Mr. Right and Mr. Wrong." To my knowledge, neuroscience has not yet detected an OrgasOMeter for mate selection.

SSRIs and other antidepressants are prescribed a lot because SSRIs made a dramatic improvement in quality of life for many people. Doctors don't give them because they want to make you worse. So please, don't see a nonmedical practitioner if you feel depressed. See a real doctor!

## Conclusion

While the facts in *True Love* are as up to date and current as possible, I don't believe this is the final version of our understanding of love. As science advances, our understanding will continue to advance, and I've included the following appendixes with that in mind. The book will hopefully continue to evolve with time and continuous feedback from readers and scientists alike.

My goals in writing *True Love* are lofty, but I believe they are achievable. I hope *True Love* will help those who read it to avoid the increasingly common love-related problems described in the book. I hope it will help many to achieve better love lives and more joy from love. I hope it will help some to accept genetic differences that cannot be changed in their mate. I hope it will help guide all who read it to seek love the correct way, with knowledge of the physical processes involved in seeking, finding, and keeping True Love.

FRED NOUR
November 2016

# ACKNOWLEDGMENTS

First and foremost, I must thank my wife, not only for helping me feel how wonderful True Love can be, but also for her patience and support during the time when I was very busy with my second wife, this book.

I am indebted to all my patients who had the courage to share with me the intimate details of their lives and their feelings about love.

I am very grateful to everybody at Niguel Publishing for all the work they did on my book. Their wonderful professionals made *True Love* the quality book I dreamed of.

I want to express my gratitude to all the professionals who helped produce this book. I wish to thank Dr. John Ellis for his input on the neuroscience behind True Love.

Thanks also to the artists whose pictures and illustrations were available to me to include in this book, including Adobe Stock, Dreamtime, Wikidoc.org, John Wiley & Sons, Elsevier, the US Department of Health and Human Services, the National Academy of Sciences, and the Mayo Foundation.

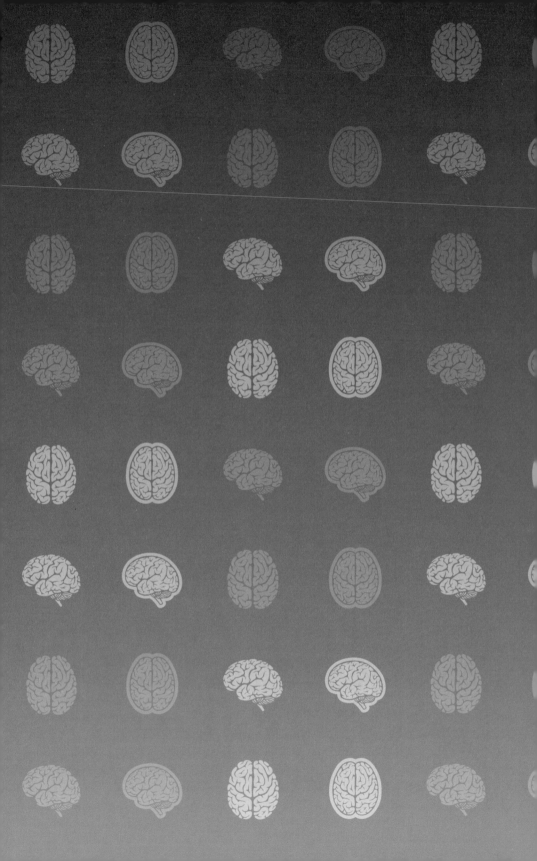

# APPENDIXES

---

In the Conclusion, I stated my goals for writing *True Love*, which I decided to do while knowing how difficult it can be to make the necessarily complex science easy for the everyday reader to understand. From the many lectures I've given to the public over the years, I've learned that most people want to understand general concepts and facts about our body, but naturally are bored with deep or intricate scientific details. My goals in writing meant that I had to decide how best to present these facts and ideas to readers.

I had two options. I could write a scientifically proven, data-driven book on the study of love. That would most likely bore the nonacademic reader, but would be of interest to scientists and researchers. The other option was to write an easy-to-read version with minimal scientific jargon, which everybody could enjoy and learn from. *True Love* uses this second approach, so it's not meant to be a scientific research paper or a thesis about the science of love. (There will be a future edition written specifically for scientists and psychologists.) Those in search of detailed description and well-researched facts will still find them inside *True Love*'s pages, and in the following appendixes.

The first appendix goes more in depth about brain chemicals and their relation to love. Most people are quite happy to know that there are certain systems in their brain that perceive this or that, but don't care where exactly these cells are located in the brain. Those who want to know more will find that here. The second appendix includes what I promised to give—a thorough discussion of the recent controversy about the accuracy of the fMRI.

– FN

# THE LIMBIC BRAIN & LOVE
# CHEMICALS SUMMARY

---

## Love Chemicals Summary

| Family | Children | Grandchildren | Functions |
|---|---|---|---|
| Monoamines | Catecholamines | Epinephrine | Fear, negative feelings |
| | | | Paranoia, jealousy |
| | | | Tachycardia (fast heartbeat) |
| | | | Long-term memory recall |
| | | | Shakiness, anxiety, sweating |
| | | Norepinephrine | Loss of sleep |
| | | | More attention |
| | | | Tachycardia |
| | | | ANS activity |
| | | | Mate selection: Focus on one mate, ignore the rest |
| | | | Coordinates the activity of 3 brain parts |
| | | | Connects limbic brain to new brain |
| | | | PFC makes decisions |
| | | | OFC enhances risk |
| | | | OFC causes addiction behavior, risks |

*(continued on next page)*

| Family | Children | Grandchildren | Functions |
|---|---|---|---|
| Monoamines | Catecholamines | Norepinephrine | ACC enhances caution |
| | | | ACC links NB & ILB, mate selection influence |
| | | | Enhances nonapeptides NE; prepares for true love |
| | | | Appetite center (up) via increase dopamine |
| | | | Social emotional response |
| | | | ? responsible for fantasia |
| | | | Dopamine modulation |
| | | | Serotonin modulation |
| | | | Suppression of bad choices (mates) |
| | | | Sympathetic activation: Dilated pupils Sweating |
| | | Dopamine | Movements (such as automatic walking) |
| | | | Joys and pleasures, euphoria |
| | | | Addictions Gene dependent (tryptophan hydroxylase type 2, serotonin enzyme) |
| | | | Sex drive & orgasm (SDN) |
| | | | Illusions |
| | | | Delusions |
| | | | Confused thinking |
| | | | Pair bonding |
| | Serotonin | Serotonin *receptor number in parenthesis* | Modulates dopamine … (1a) … in PFC |
| | | | Sex drive, by dopamine on SDN |
| Monoamines | Serotonin | Serotonin | Modulates nonapeptides (increasing bonding) |

| Family | Children | Grandchildren | Functions |
|---|---|---|---|
| | | | Modulates norepinephrine (2a) |
| | | | Memory recall (1a) |
| | | | Anxiety / depression gets better (1a) |
| | | | Depression gets worse (2c) |
| | | | Appetite up (2c) |
| | | | Vomiting (3) |
| | | | Hallucinations (1a suppresses, 2a increases it) |
| | | | Sleep maintenance |
| | | | OCD suppressed by 5HT |
| | | | Addictions |
| | | | Compulsion and obsession |
| | | | Hoarding (compulsion) |
| Nonapeptdes | Oxytocin | | More estrogen receptors |
| | | | Needs norepinephrine |
| | | | Decreases aggression |
| | Vasopressin | | More testosterone receptors |
| | | | Increases aggression |
| | Both Oxytocin & Pitocin | | Social recognition |
| | | | Social bonding |
| | | | Pair bonding |
| | | | Monogamy |
| | | | Bonding and identification |
| | | | Trust |
| | | | Passion |
| | | | Harmonious relationships |
| | | | Changed in perception of partner |

## Partial List of Intermediate Limbic Brain Centers

For each center, there is one center in the right brain and one in the left brain. Sometimes these have different functions between the sides of the brain.

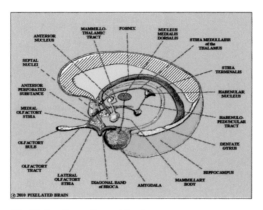

*Limbic brain centers, side view*

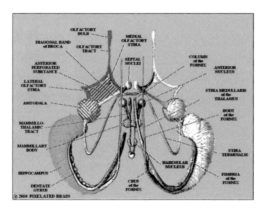

*Limbic brain centers, top view*

# The Hypothalamus

The hypothalamus is the "central command center" of the limbic system.

It controls most of the functions in the intermediate limbic brain system.

It's about the size of an almond in human adults.

Like a military's central command center, the hypothalamus is relatively small but controls many divisions and coordinates all the action over the big defense forces (army, navy, air force, and so on).

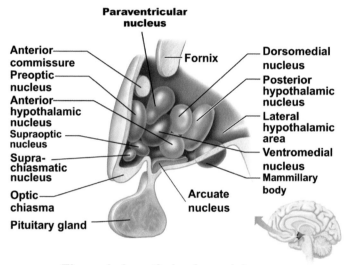

**The main hypothalamic nuclei.**

*The hypothalamic nuclei*

*The Anatomical Classification of Hypothalamic Centers and Some of Their Functions.*

| Region | Nucleus | Function | Comments |
|---|---|---|---|
| **Anterior Area** | Medial PreOptic Area (MPOA) | Sexually Dimorphic Nucleus | Male vs. female behavior = proceptive and receptive behavior |
| | | Gonadotropin release hormones by SDN | Stimulates release of sex hormones from testis and ovary |
| | | Maternal behavior | Bonding and caring for offspring |
| | Supraoptic Nucleus | Oxytocin release, Vasopressin release | True love inducing chemicals |
| | Para-ventricular Nucleus | Thyrotropin releasing hormone release | Increases thyroid function = stimulates metabolism |
| | | Corticotrophin releasing hormone | Stress response in body induces parturition, cortisol release |
| | | Somatostatin release | Inhibits growth hormone Inhibits glucose metabolism |
| | Anterior Hypothalamic Nucleus | Thermoregulation (Median POA) | Controls body temperature |
| | | Panting | Stimulates heavy breathing |
| | | Sweating | Temperature lowering |
| | | Thyrotropin inhibition | Suppresses metabolism |
| | Supra-chiasmatic Nucleus | Circadian rhythms | Our internal 24-hour clock |
| **Tuberal Area** | Dorso-Medial Nucleus | Blood pressure | Controls blood pressure |
| | | Heart rate | Controls heart rate |
| | | GI stimulation | Increases intestinal activity |
| | Ventro-Medial Nucleus | Satiety center | Suppresses appetite for food and sex |
| | | Neuro-endocrine control | Controls the release of hormones from the endocrine systems |

| Region | Nucleus | Function | Comments |
|--------|---------|----------|----------|
| **Tuberal Area** | Arcuate Nucleus | Growth hormone releasing hormone | Releases growth hormone causing growth in body size |
| | | Feeding | Stimulate eating |
| | | Dopamine mediated prolactin inhibition | Stops lactation |
| **Posterior Area** | Posterior Nucleus | Increase blood pressure | Raises blood pressure |
| | | Pupillary dilatation | Makes pupils bigger |
| | | Shivering | Heat production, can cause fever |
| | | Vasopressin release | True love inducing chemicals |
| | Mamillary bodies | Memory | Recent and old memory storage and recall |
| **Lateral Area** | Tubero-Mamillary Nucleus | Appetite (feeding behavior) | Orexin control |
| | | Arousal (wakefulness) | Awake and alert vs. sleepy and lethargic, coma if no arousal at all |
| | | Pain inhibition | Stops pain |
| | | Blood pressure regulation | Regulate blood pressure |
| | | Thermal and energy regulation | Regulate body temperature and energy control? Anorexia, obesity related |
| | | Visceral regulation | Irritable bowel syndrome seems related to overactivity here |
| | Ventro Lateral Preoptic area (VLPA) | Non-REM sleep regulation | Dysfunction here causes sleep disorders, insomnia, narcolepsy. |
| | | Arousal (wakefulness) | Some drugs (anesthetics) work on this area |

# APPENDIX B

# HOW WE STUDY THE FUNCTIONS OF THE BRAIN, AND HOW FUNCTIONAL MAGNETIC RESONANCE IMAGING WORKS

---

Why have studies based on fMRI imaging recently been questioned?

Before delving into the recent findings about functional MRI (fMRI) usefulness, it's a good idea to give a brief overview of the common methods used to study brain functions today. My thoughts and the recent findings about the fMRI's place as a useful tool (or not) begins after this section.

## Methods Medical Doctors Use to Study Brain Functions

The purpose of this section is to familiarize you with some of the common methods currently used to study brain functions. No one method used alone can tell us everything. In fact, we typically use multiple methods, each one telling us one aspect of function. You need not remember any of this. It's just given to help you recognize the diversity of methods used.

### Autopsies on Humans and Animals

This time-honored method started millennia ago, and by 1858, when *Gray's Anatomy* was published, we knew the details of our internal body structures. Further examination of structures evolved with more precise technologies. We can now see minor cell details under the electron microscope. Various staining techniques help identify certain structures by staining them with certain colored dyes.

## Experiments on Living Animals[12]

To the surprise of many, we share about 90 percent of our genetic code with animals. Animal studies have contributed a tremendous amount of knowledge about our biology and the biology of love. Via the study of animal behaviors, we can record the chemicals associated with different behaviors. We can block the effect of certain chemicals and see the behavioral effect on animals. We can increase (stimulate) the effect of certain chemicals and see the effect on animal behavior. We can insert tiny tubes to measure chemicals and so on. A good part of the knowledge in this book was drawn from animal studies.

## Neuropharmacology

Our behaviors are based on the effects of multiple neurotransmitters. We can give medication or pharmaceutical agents to enhance or block these neurotransmitters and see the effect on behaviors. A very significant amount of knowledge in humans was acquired by this method. This is done on living humans and is an excellent way to understand human behavior.

## Neurophysiology

These are electrical studies of the brain.

### EEG: Electroencephalogram

There are rhythmic generators in the brain that produce electric firing of other brain cells. The *electric-voltage* fluctuations are recorded by multiple voltmeters and graphed on paper or digital files. These records are analyzed by a neurologist for significance. The EEG is most useful for evaluating seizures, since these are caused by abnormal electric signals in the brain.

---

12. Sorry, animal activists, for any offense. I personally do not do animal research.

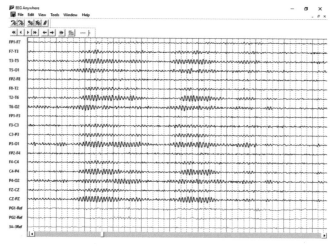

*EEG*

## MEG: Magnetoencephalography

EEG measures *voltage* changes between two points on the brain surface from the travel of electricity. Any electrical *current* in the brain will produce a *magnetic field*, and it's this field that is measured by the magnet used in MEG. Combining both EEG and MEG gives a better image of the electrical changes in the brain.

### Visual Evoked Response

This is done by sending a visual stimulus to the eye and recording the time it takes to reach the visual area in the brain. This measures the health of this pathway.

### Auditory Evoked Response

This is done by sending sound (clicks) and recording the electric-current fields generated. Five waves are generated at five different locations in the brain, mainly in the lower brain. The time difference between the waves measures the health of that segment. This is used to localize points of dysfunction in this conduction system.

## Brain Mapping

Brain mapping is the science of generating visual images of the brain structures. This is a partial list, since the options keep expanding.

### CAT Scan: Computerized Axial Tomography or CT Scan

This test came into use in 1972. The CAT scan uses X-rays and a computer program to generate 3-D images of the brain. Because X-rays don't penetrate bone well, the thick human skull makes the base of the brain hard to see. MRI shows the brain better because it can't see bone well.

### Perfusion CT

This is a CT that measures the blood flow in the brain, called perfusion of the brain. However, its findings appear more consistent than fMRI. It is commonly used to look at blood flow during acute strokes.

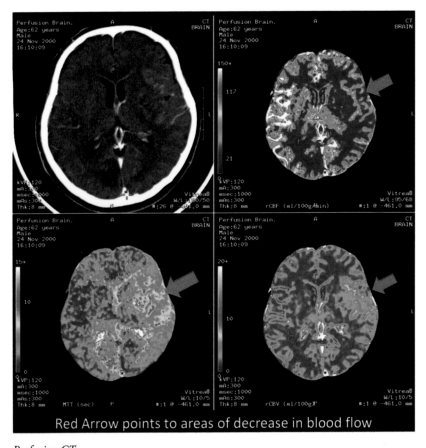

Red Arrow points to areas of decrease in blood flow

*Perfusion CT*

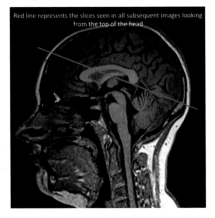

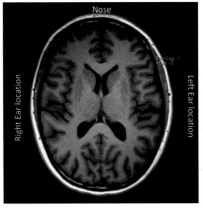

Side view of MRI of the brain          Top view of MRI of the brain

### MRI: Magnetic Resonance Imaging

This technique uses a magnetic field, radio waves, and an electric-field gradient to generate 3-D images of the brain. The MRI is of tremendous value in studying the structure of the brain, because we can see fairly finely detailed images of the brain's superficial and deep structures. The technique was discovered in 1977 and came into popular use in medicine in the 1980s. It's now the gold standard in seeing the brain's internal structures. It's very safe to use; no harm has been ever proven from it.

### Diffusion MRI

The diffusion-weighted MRI measures the motion of water molecules in tissues. It's the earliest way to visualize an acute brain injury, such as a stroke.

### FLAIR MRI: Fluid-Attenuated Inversion Recovery Images

This technology allows better visualization of deep structures near the brain's center.

## Susceptibility MRI or SWI (Susceptibility Weighted Imaging)

This image uses the distortion of the local magnetic field by the movement of magnetically charged particles and is useful in detecting blood products, calcium, iron, and similar elements. These show as black dots on a white background. This technique is also used to generate fMRI images.

## MRS: Magnetic Resonance Spectroscopy

This is a variant of MRI. It selects a small area of the brain and then measures the levels of metabolic products in this small area. MRS is used to estimate the metabolic activity in this small area of the brain. As an example, a patient comes in with a seizure, and his routine MRI shows a small abnormal area in the brain, but we don't know its nature. MRS can assess if this area is hypermetabolic, and thus likely a tumor or infection, or hypometabolic, and thus most likely a section of dead tissue from a silent stroke.

## fMRI: Functional MRI

This was invented in 1990 at Bell Labs. This is a traditional MRI with overlapping, colored, susceptibility MRI images from changes in oxygenation at a specific location. It depends on blood-oxygen-level

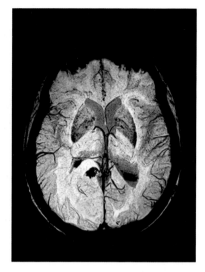

Susceptibility MRI

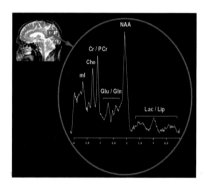

MRS

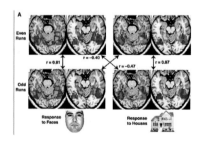

fMRI. This image purportedly shows brain reaction to looking at faces versus buildings.

dependent signals, known as BOLD, and presumably measures changes in oxygen levels at a specific location. It does *not* measure neuronal activity. It's a very slow scan because of the slow processing of the blood-oxygen-level dependent signals. Thus it can't measure very fast events in the brain. We know that increased activity at a specific brain location can increase oxygen consumption by a maximum of 5 percent. This extremely small change causes multiple technical problems. It tends to generate false positive results.

### SPECT Scan: Single-Photon Emission Computerized Tomography

This scan uses a gamma ray–emitting radioisotope that binds to certain receptors on brain cells. It uses a special camera called a gamma camera to generate pictures on top of a CT scan image.

### PET: Positive Emission Topography

This is similar to a SPECT scan in concept. Positive emission topography tracers emit positrons that produce two gamma photons to be emitted in opposite directions. A PET scanner detects these emissions' "coincidence" in time, which provides more localization information. It gives off radiation, which limits its potential.

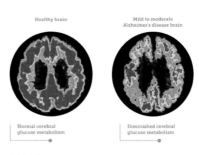

*PET Scan*

### TMS: Transcranial Magnetic Stimulation

Transcranial magnetic stimulation (TMS) is a magnetic method used to stimulate small regions of the brain. During a TMS procedure, a magnetic field generator, or "coil," is placed near the head of the person receiving the treatment. The coil produces small electric currents in the region of the brain just under it.

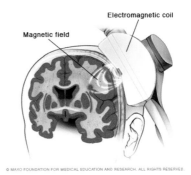

*TMS*

TMS is used to measure the connection between the brain and a muscle, to evaluate brain damage location in different diseases.

Interestingly, TMS seems promising in treating depression.

### VNS: Vagal Nerve Stimulation

The vagal nerve comes out from the lower brain to send commands to the heart, lungs, intestines, and other areas of the abdomen. It has no pain fibers; thus, its stimulation is painless. The nerve seems to suppress some brain activity, and in fact, VNS is used to suppress seizures, and it seems to help with depression. It's being studied in connection with many other disorders, too many to list here.

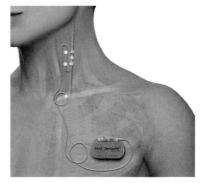

*Vagal nerve stimulation*

### DBS: Deep Brain Stimulation

This is a neurosurgical procedure invented in 1987. The procedure, done awake or under anesthesia, involves a tiny wire or multiple wires that are inserted into a specific location or locations deep in the brain. The other end of the wire is connected to a stimulator: a pacemaker, to interfere in cell activity electrically. This procedure has been of tremendous value in understanding the deep structures of the brain and is also of great therapeutic value in many brain disorders. It has revolutionized the treatment of medication-resistant Parkinson's disease, benign familial tremors, dystonia, and obsessive-compulsive disorder, and there are numerous studies ongoing for its use in brain disorders such as depression, PTSD, and chronic pain syndromes.

### DTI or DTMRI: Diffusion Tensor Imaging

This technology came into use in 1993. This is an MRI technique measuring the rate and direction

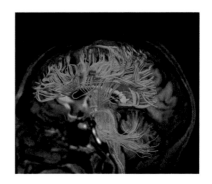

*DTI*

of water movement to generate images of the electrical cables running across different areas of the brain. This test has been of tremendous value for neurosurgeons in planning surgery on brain tumors and other abnormalities in the brain, since it gives them an individualized picture of these cables so they don't accidently injure the cables during surgery, making neurosurgery much safer.

### DaT: Dopamine Transporter Scan

This was FDA approved in 2011 and is the best way we have today to see dopamine in the brain. Dopamine is used, then taken back into the cell by a *dopamine transporter*. The DaT scan uses a radioactive substance that generates images of the transporter protein. This shows us the number of dopamine cells in the brain. It's of tremendous value in diagnosing dopamine-related disorders such as Parkinson's disease.

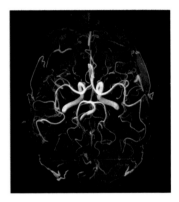

### MRA: Magnetic Resonance Angiogram

MRA is a non invasive way to see the blood vessels inside the brain while a person is awake. We can use it to detect aneurysms, blockages in vessels, and inflammation in vessel walls.

*MRA*

• • •

Many more technologies are available, but I won't mention all of them here.

> *There is an expansive array of technologies used to study brain structure (brain mapping) and function.*

Most likely, a few of them will someday play a role in helping science solve "the mystery of love" at all its phases.

In the next section, I'll return to one of these technologies—the functional MRI—and discuss information recently come to light that makes the fMRI, and most previous publications using the fMRI, less trustworthy as information sources.

# Are fMRI Scans the Best Way to Study Brain Chemistry?

Since we're nearing the last part of the book, please allow me to dig deeper into the neuroscience and debate the science behind studying love in more scientific detail.

As we just mentioned, brain imaging is called *brain mapping*. This includes CAT (computerized axial tomography), several forms of MRI (magnetic resonance imaging) including the fMRI (functional MRI), and many more technologies.

One test was relied upon in many best-selling books, such as *The Anatomy of Love* by anthropologist Helen Fisher. These books draw, sometimes quite heavily, from the results of functional MRI (fMRI) brain mapping.

The test is now over twenty-six years old and is one of many technologies we have today to study the function of the brain while we're alive. fMRI combines two of these technologies, namely *traditional MRI image* and MRI-based *susceptibility image*.

The scandal about this form of MRI climaxed recently, and questions about these technologies peaked. These newly reported questions about the test's validity have the potential to affect those who have learned about love from these fMRI studies in the past and made decisions based solely, or even primarily, upon belief that the fMRI had given accurate data.

To understand the problems with relying on these images, first let's look at the concepts behind fMRI. This will help us decide whether fMRI is a remarkable feat of modern technology or not.

## Concept One in fMRI Science

There are well-defined *networks* of brain cells: the dopamine network, the serotonin network, and others. Each network is composed of multiple members connected together by axons (tiny electric wires), that work sequentially, independent of other networks. A signal starts in a cell at one end and spreads to the next member cell, then the next member cell, and so on. This is like a football game where Player A uses energy to catch the ball and throw it to Player B, who also increases his metabolism to catch the ball and send it to the next player, and so on. Each cell will *increase* its activity to respond to the signal from the previous cell member and to send it to the next cell member of that well-defined network. This is known as *cell activation*.

## Concept Two in fMRI Science

These networks are inactive at rest. This is called *default mode*, and the network is called the *default mode network*, DMN for short. This is a resting, fixed, low-level metabolic activity against which we measure all other activities. This is like comparing your metabolism when asleep and then when awake and active. We should expect the metabolic activity to lessen during sleep and increase with waking-state activities. Thus with mental activity, this default-mode metabolism increases in actively working cells—the cells are *metabolically active* or "activated."

## Concept Three in fMRI Science

Brain cells don't store any oxygen. As the brain cell becomes more active, it needs more energy, and thus more oxygen. The blood flow increases in the cell's active area in reaction to increased metabolism to provide needed oxygen. The oxygen is taken from oxyhemoglobin (oxygen attached to hemoglobin) in the blood. This converts oxyhemoglobin to deoxyhemoglobin (*de*= take away, *oxy*= oxygen). With the loss of oxygen (two negative charges), deoxyhemoglobin becomes positively charged. In a magnetic field, positive and negative particles move in opposite directions in relation to the magnetic pole. This change of direction is detected in the susceptibility images. The word *susceptibility* came from the Latin word *susceptibilis*, meaning "to take up" or "to capture." In science, susceptibility indicates whether a material is attracted into or repelled out of a magnetic field. We can generate pictures of any magnetically charged chemicals in the brain based on their movements in relationship to the magnet. The susceptibility image could be color-coded with any colors desired. This image could be superimposed on the routine MRI image in any color your heart desires, creating the fMRI images.

This generated signal is called the BOLD (blood-oxygen-level dependent) signal. This signal reflects the decrease in oxygen from its use by active cells.

Last, please note that fMRI doesn't prove that a certain chemical is released, but it *assumes* that, based on the type of cells usually present at a specific location in the brain.

Now that we understand the basic concepts behind fMRI, we can move on to analyze the problems with them one by one.

## Problems with Concept One in fMRI Science

*Networks are independent of each other.*
As a neurologist, I know that all systems are dynamically balanced and connected all the time. If a patient has Parkinson's disease from the reduced release of dopamine, I can treat him by increasing his dopamine brain release. However, if the patient can't tolerate the dopamine-increasing medications, we can get the same effect by blocking a different network, the acetylcholine network. We get the same result by affecting either system.

*Each network is composed of multiple members connected together by axons (tiny electric wires), and works sequentially.*

Children, say at eight years of age, don't have the connection between these centers developed yet, a lack of connection caused by the axons being *unmyelinated*, like copper wires without the plastic coating. However, these children are able to do the same type of thinking and feeling as adults. Their fMRI images look similar to fMRI images in adults who have these connections developed. This questions the concept of the default mode network, of which its proponents claim that the activity is based on connections between the cells in the network.

## Problems with Concept Two in fMRI Science

The baseline activity is that which reflects the network's basic metabolic energy needs. With activity, these networks increase their metabolic needs and consume more oxygen, which fMRI believers call *activation*. They believe that a decrease in oxygen consumption below the normal resting level happens, and they call this *deactivation*.

We have evidence that the default networks consume *more* energy at rest than while doing a range of explicit tasks. Mental activity should *decrease* the oxygen consumption, causing less blood-oxygen-level dependent signal to reveal itself on an fMRI, not an increase (activation).

If the resting state of the default mode network is the baseline of metabolic function, how can the brain function with less energy during deactivation?

## Problems with Concept Three in fMRI Science

*The BOLD (blood-oxygen-level dependent) signal reflects the decrease in oxygen levels from its use by active cells.*

It's proven that merely changing one's breathing pattern, without doing any thinking or any mental activity at all, changes the fMRI blood-oxygen-level dependent signals, both baseline metabolic activity and the metabolic activity associated with mental tasks known as activation tasks. Do you feel more love for your mate when you breathe faster or when you breathe slower? Or are you like me—I never feel any difference in my love by changing my breathing pattern.

It appears that the fMRI signal is dependent on blood flow and not on metabolic activity in the cell. We change the brain blood flow in comatose patients by changing the breathing pattern on their ventilators.

We know that certain locations in the brain are more susceptible to certain pathology than others; for example, a drop in oxygen causes more brain injury in certain locations than others. Could the difference in signal be from the difference in normal cell metabolic activity? Thus, could the default mode changes be associated with the normal variation of metabolic activity?

fMRI images measure an average of twenty seconds of activity. Does our brain function that slowly? Do you spend twenty seconds to just look at an image? I personally review slideshows on my computer at the rate of three to four seconds for each image. Are we including another sixteen or seventeen seconds of other activities in the brain? Which of the twenty seconds are we actually measuring?

## Problems with the "Brain at Rest Consumes Less Energy" Concept

You should expect baseline metabolic needs stay the same all the time. If you put people under anesthesia and stimulate their vision using goggles with lights, you get a *bigger* blood-oxygen-level dependent signal while there is no increase in brain-cell activity, since they're unconscious: under anesthesia, maybe there is a decrease in the BOLD signal.

Many question the concept, "The brain does nothing unless it's instructed to." That's like saying that we do nothing unless we receive a bill, and only then will we start working. If this was the case, nobody should ever have savings. We know without doubt that all neurotransmitters are premade and stored in nerve terminals (in *vesicles*). These neurotransmitters are released when the electric signal reaches the nerve terminal. The neurotransmitters aren't made the moment we need them. Just like earning money, you work all the time, but you save the money and spend it only when you need to; we consume more energy working than spending money. This matches the brain's increased energy consumption at rest and less consumption with activity.

It's been proven that many decreases in function, which fMRI enthusiasts call *deactivation*, happen independent from the task. Four different areas have shown this deactivation, regardless of whether or not you're doing a mental task.

Areas of *activation* and *deactivation* in the brain aren't consistent in all studies for the same task. fMRIs that measure oxygen use, and PET scans that measure glucose metabolism, show identical images to task activation. However, there's no evidence that the oxygen consumption has any temporal relationship to glucose consumption.

*The signal in fMRI must have another source, probably a neurophysiologic and not a neurocognitive (thinking) source.*

If an fMRI signal suggests an internal thought process, why do we do the same when we pay passive attention to the external environment? We still get *activation* and *deactivation* signals.

In a study on rats' brain signals, while navigating a maze the rats showed the changes of *activation* and *deactivation* as they navigated the maze. However, when they stopped the navigation, the *activation* and *deactivation* continued even though they weren't doing any mental processing!

Further criticism: The fMRI images use *subtraction* of the activation signal from baseline activity. Flaws and fallacies in subtraction have been debated by many scientists. The international radiology encyclopedia Radiopaedia.org (http://radiopaedia.org/articles/functional-mri) states, "fMRI is technically challenging to perform as the techniques used to visualize cortical activity (typically BOLD imaging) rely on *minute* changes in a low signal-to-noise ratio (SNR) environment." Basically they're saying that it's difficult and unreliable to try to listen to loudness changes of a whisper in a very noisy environment. You can use this type of imaging to check the surface of the brain, the *cortex*, but not the deep structures in the brain, such as the ventral tegmental area.

The continuous recording of OEF (oxygen extraction fraction, the amount of oxygen taken from blood) continuously fluctuates, suggesting that these cells are in a dynamic state and not a fixed baseline.

## The History of the Scandal about fMRI Studies

- 1990: fMRI was discovered. Many studies started using it to study cognition, emotions, and personality.
- 1994: A mere four years after the discovery, neurologist Karl Friston and colleagues in London published a paper about problems in fMRI data analysis: "The probability that one or more activated regions of a specified volume, or larger, could have occurred by chance." This was mainly ignored.
- 2009: Massachusetts Institute of Technology (MIT) and the University of California in San Diego looked at the statistical methods used in analysis of fMRI studies. They requested the raw (initial unprocessed) data from fMRI researchers. Only about 50 percent of researchers submitted their data. Some submitted just one of many studies. MIT analysis revealed that 25 to 40 percent of the studies used wrong statistical methods, resulting in the report, "Puzzlingly High Correlations in fMRI Studies of Emotion, Personality and Social Cognition." http://www.pashler.com/Articles/Vul_etal_2008inpress.pdf
- 2009: In one real but satirical fMRI study, a salmon was shown pictures of humans in different emotional states. The authors provided evidence, according to two different commonly used statistical methods, of areas in the salmon's brain suggesting meaningful activity. It could easily be concluded that the salmon perceived and interacted with human facial expressions. The big problem was that the salmon was dead. It had been purchased by the researcher the morning of the experiment from a fish market. http://prefrontal.org/files/posters/Bennett-Salmon-2009.pdf

- This study was awarded the notorious and farcical-minded IgNobel Prize. http://www.improbable.com/ig/winners/
- The story was reported in *Scientific American*. http://blogs.scientificamerican.com/scicurious-brain/ignobel-prize-in-neuroscience-the-dead-salmon-study/
- 2010: Dr. Russ Poldrack at Stanford University started an Open fMRI Repository for scientists to store and share their research data so others could look at and reanalyze them if needed. Not all researchers participated.
- 2013: Sally Satel, MD published a book entitled *Brainwashed: The Seductive Appeal of Mindless Neuroscience*, basically criticizing the deception of fMRI reports: "You've seen the headlines: This is your brain in love. Or God. Or envy. Or happiness. And they're reliably accompanied by articles boasting pictures of color-drenched brains." Satel criticized the rise of "neuromarketing" and profiteering from the marketing of neuroscience.
  - Book review in *Huffington Post* http://www.huffingtonpost.com/dj-jaffe/brainwashed-the-seductive_b_3712860.html
  - Article in *Time* magazine http://ideas.time.com/2013/05/30/dont-read-too-much-into-brain-scans/
- 2016: The most prestigious medical journal is *Proceedings of the National Academy of Sciences* (PNAS). The National Academy of Science was founded by President Abraham Lincoln in 1863 as "advisors to the nation on science." Membership in the Academy is by invitation only. Of just over 2,000 members, nearly 200 are Nobel Prize winners.

  The July 12, 2016 issue of *PNAS* reported a study by Swedish scientists looking at fMRI software: "Cluster failure: Why fMRI inferences for spatial extent have inflated false-positive rates." The authors examined the three most commonly used fMRI software programs, used by 80 percent of researchers, using data from the Open fMRI Repository at Stanford University. The Swedish researchers conducted three million task-group analyses of fMRI data, using the data of people at rest (null data) who weren't engaged in any cognitive activity. Scientifically, these brain images should show no activity on fMRI scans. They discovered that over 70 percent of images showed false-positive correlation. The conclusion: "These results question the validity of many of the 40,000 fMRI studies."

- 2016: On July, 15, the esteemed journal *Science* reported on the study in its "News in depth" section: "Brain scans are prone to false positives, study says. Common software settings may have skewed the statistics for thousands of studies." http://www.sciencemagazinedigital.org/sciencemagazine/15_july_2016_Main?sub_id=UI36dy9C7O4Y&u1=41481570&folio=232&pg=16#pg16

- 2016: On July 5, the journal *Nature*, after knowing about the Swedish study, announced that "*Nature* promotes research data sharing," and set new criteria for doing so. *Nature* wanted to prevent similar flawed studies in their most prestigious journal. http://blogs.nature.com/ofschemesandmemes/2016/07/05/promoting-research-data-sharing-at-springer-nature

What you need to consider, based on my opinions, as both a reader of this book and as a medical consumer, are the following two statements:

*The fMRI is not the best way to see the functions inside the brain.*

*The fMRI is based on questionable science.*

# BIBLIOGRAPHY

Algoe, Sara B., and Baldwin M. Way. "Evidence for a role of the oxytocin system, indexed by genetic variation in CD38, in social bonding effects of expressed gratitude." *Social Cognitive and Affective Neuroscience Advance Access.* (January 5, 2014): 1–34.

Allendorf, K., and Dirgha G. "Determinants of marital quality in an arranged marriage society." *Social Science Research.* (January, 2013): 42, no. 159–70.

Aragona, B. J., Yan Liu, Y. Joy Yu, J. T. Curtis, J. M. Detwiler, T. R. Insel, and Z. Wang. "Nucleus accumbens dopamine differentially mediates the formation and maintenance of monogamous pair bonds." *Nature Neuroscience.* (Published online: December 4, 2005): 9(1): 133–139. | doi:10.1038/nn1613.

Arai, A., Y. Hirota, N. Miyase, S. Miyata, L. J. Young, Y. Osako, K. Yuri, and S. Mitsui. "A single prolonged stress paradigm produces enduring impairments in social bonding in monogamous prairie voles." *Behavioural Brain Research.* (Epub August 10, 2016): 315:83-93. doi:10.1016/j.bbr.2016.08.022.

Argiolas A., and M. R. Melis. "The neurophysiology of the sexual cycle." *Journal of Endocrinological Investigation.* (2003): 26 (3Suppl): 20–2.

Aston-Jones G., and J. D. Cohen. "An Integrative Theory of Locus Coeruleus-Norepinephrine Function: Adaptive Gain and Optimal Performance." *Annual Review of Neuroscience.* (2005): 28: 403–450.

Aston-Jones, G., and B. Waterhouse. "Locus Coeruleus: From global projection system to adaptive regulation of behavior." *Brain Research.* (Mar 9, 2016): 1645 75–78. doi: 10.1016/j.brainres.2016.03.001.

Auger, A. P., J. M. Meredith, G. L. Snyder, and J. D. Blaustein. "Estradiol increases phosphorylation of a dopamine and cyclic AMP-regulated phosphoprotein (DARPP-32) in female rat brain." *Journal of Neuroendocrinology.* (2001): 13, 761–768.

Bakerville, T. A., J. Allard, C. Wayman, and A. J. Douglas. "Dopamine-Oxytocin interactions in penile erection." *The European Journal of Neuroscience.* (2009): 30: 2151–64. doi: 10.1111/j.1460-9568.2009.06999.x.

Bartz, J. A., J. Zaki, N. Bolger, and K. N. Oschner. "Social effects of oxytocin in humans: Context and person matter." *Trends in Cognitive Sciences.* (2011): 15(7):301–309. doi: 10.1016/j.tics.2011.05.002.

Baum, M. J., B. J. Everitt, J. Herbert, and E. B. Keverne. "Hormonal basis of proceptivity and receptivity in female primates." *Archives of Sexual Behavior.* (May, 1977): 6(3): 173–92.

Becker, J. B., C. N. Rudick, and W. J. Jenkins. "The role of dopamine in the nucleus accumbens and striatum during sexual behavior in the female rat." *The Journal of Neuroscience.* (May 1, 2001): 21(9), 3236–3241.

Belluz, J., B. Plumer, and B. Resnick. September 7, 2016. *Vox,* "The 7 biggest problems facing science, according to 270 scientists." http://www.vox.com/2016/7/14/12016710/science-challeges-research-funding-peer-review-process.

Bennett, C. M., A. A. Baird, M. B. Miller, and George L. Wolford. "Neural correlates of interspecies perspective taking in the post-mortem Atlantic Salmon: An argument for multiple comparisons correction." http://prefrontal.org/files/posters/Bennett-Salmon-2009.pdf.

Berridge, C. W., and B. D. Waterhouse. "The locus coeruleus-noradrenergic system: modulation of behavioral state and state-dependent cognitive processes." *Brain Research, Brain Research Reviews.* (2003): Apr; 42(1): 33–84.

Bester-Meredith J. K., L. J. Young, and C. A. Marler. "Species differences in paternal behavior and aggression in Perimysium and their associations with vasopressin immunoreactivity and receptors." *Hormones and Behavior.* (August, 1999): 36 (1), 25–38.

Booth, T. C., M. Nathan, A. D. Waldman, A. M. Quigley, A. H. Schapira, and J. Buscombe. "The Role of Functional Dopamine-Transporter SPECT imaging in Parkinsonian Syndromes, Part 1." *American Journal of Neuroradiology.* (February, 2015): 36 (2): 229–35. doi: 10.3174/ajnr.A3970.

Buckner, R. L., and J. L. Vincent. "Unrest at rest: Default activity and spontaneous network correlations." *NeuroImage.* (2007): 37 1091–1096.

Buckner, R. L., J. R. Andrews-Hanna, and D. L. Schacter. "The brain's default network: Anatomy, function, and relevance to disease." *Annals of the New York Academy of Sciences.* (March, 2008): 1124: 1–38. doi: 10.1196/annals.1440.011.

Burkett, J. P., and L. J. Young. "The behavioral, anatomical and pharmacological parallels between social attachment, love and addiction." *Psychopharmacology (Berl).* (2012): 224(1): 1–26.

Burri, A., M. Heinrichs, M. Schedlowski, and T. H. Kruger. "The acute effects of intranasal oxytocin administration on endocrine and sexual function in males." *Psychoneuroendocrinology.* (2008): 33, 591–600.

Buss, D. M., et al. "International preferences in selecting mates: A study of 37 societies." *Journal of Cross-Cultural Psychology.* (1990): 21, 5–47.

Caldwell, H. K., H. Lee, A. H. Macbeth, and W. S. Young. "Vasopressin: Behavioral roles of an 'original' neuropeptide." *Progressive Neurobiology.* (January, 2008): 84(1): 1–24.

Canetto, S. S., and D. Lester. "Love and achievement motives in women's and men's suicide notes." *The Journal of Psychology*. (2002): 136, 573–576.

Cardinal, R. N., and N. J. Howes. "Effects of lesions of the accumbens core on choice between small uncertain rewards in rats." *BMC Neuroscience*. (2005): 6, 37–56.

Carmichael, M. S., V. L. Warburton, J. Dixen, and J. M. Davidson. "Relationship among cardiovascular, muscular, and oxytocin responses during human sexual activity." *Archives of Sexual Behavior*. (1994): 23, 59–79.

Carmichael, M. S., R. Humbert, J. Dixen, G. Palmisano, W. Greenleaf, and J. M. Davidson. "Plasma oxytocin increases in the human sexual response." *The Journal of Clinical Endocrinology and Metabolism*. (1987): 64, 27–31.

Carter, C. S., A. DeVries, S. E. Taymans, R. L. Roberts, J. R. Williams, and L. L. Getz. "Peptides, steroids, and pair-bonding. In The integrative neurobiology of affiliation, vol. 807." Edited by C. S. Carter, I. I. Lederhendler, and B. Kirkpatrick. *Annals of the New York Academy of Sciences*. (1997): 260–272.

Carter, C. S. "Neuroendocrine perspectives on social attachment and love." *Psychoneuroendocrinology*. (1998): 23, 779–818.

Carter, C. S. "Oxytocin and sexual behavior." *Neuroscience and Biobehavioral Reviews*. (1992): 1, 131–144.

Carter, C. S., H. Pournajafi-Nazarloo, K. M. Kramer, T. E. Ziegler, R. White-Traut, D. Bello, and D. Schwertz. "Oxytocin: behavioral associations and potential as a salivary biomarker." *Annals of the New York Academy of Sciences*. (2007): 1098, 312–322.

Cavanaugh, J. M., C. Huffman, A. M. Harnisch, and J. A. French. "Marmosets treated with oxytocin are more socially attractive to their long-term mate." *Frontiers in Behavioral Neuroscience*. (2015): 9: 251.

Champagne, F., J. Diorio, S. Sharma, M. J. Meaney. "Naturally occurring variations in maternal behavior in the rat are associated with differences in estrogen-inducible central oxytocin receptors." *Proceedings of the National Academy of Sciences of the United States of America*. (2001): 98, 12736–12741.

Chandler, D. J. "Evidence for a specialized role of the locus coeruleus noradrenergic system in cortical circuitry and behavioral operations." *Brain Research*. (June 15, 2016): 1641.

Chenu, F., M. El Mansari, and P. Blier. "Electrophysiological Effects of Repeated Administration of Agomelatine on the Dopamine, Norepinephrine, and Serotonin Systems in the Rat Brain." *Neuropsychopharmacology*. (2013): 38, 275–284.

Chitnis, D. "Huge increase in divorce, separation cases in Indian families in the US. Geetha Ravindra." http://www.americanbazaaronline.com/2014/03/24/huge-increase-divorce-separation-cases-indian-families-us-geetha-ravindra/.

Cho, M. M., A. C. DeVries, J. R. Williams, and C. S. Carter. "The effects of oxytocin and vasopressin on partner preferences in male and female prairie voles (Microtus ochrogaster)." *Behavioral Neuroscience*. (1999): 113, 1071–1079.

Churchland, P. S., and P. Winkielman. "Modulating social behavior with oxytocin: How does it work? What does it mean?" *Hormones and Behavior.* (2012): 61(3): 392–399.

Cilia, R., et al. "Tryptophan hydroxylase type 2 variants modulate severity and outcome of addictive behavior in Parkinson's disease." *Parkinsonism and Related Disorders.* (2016): 29, 96–103.

Corrales, E., A. Navarro, P. Cuenca, and D. Campos. "Candidate gene study reveals DRD1 and DRD2 as putative interacting risk factors for youth depression." *Psychiatry Research.* (July, 2016): 20:244: 71–77.

Cour, F., S. Droupy, et al. "Anatomy and physiology of sexuality." *Progressive Urology.* (2013 Jul):23(9): 547–61.

Cox K. H., K. M. Quinnies, et al. "Number of X-chromosome genes influences social behavior and vasopressin gene expression in mice." *Psychoneuroendocrinology.* (2015 Jan): 51: 271–81.

Cox, K. H., P. J. Bonthuisa, and E. F. Rissman. "Mouse model systems to study sex chromosome genes and behavior: Relevance to humans." *Frontiers in Neuroendocrinology.* (2014 October): 35(4): 405–419.

Cragg, S. J., M. E. Rice, and S. A. Greenfield. "Heterogeneity of Electrically Evoked Dopamine Release and Reuptake in Substantia Nigra, Ventral Tegmental Area, and Striatum." *Journal of Neurophysiology.* (1997 Feb): 77(2): 863–73.

Creutz, L. M, and M. F. Kritzer. "Estrogen receptor-beta immunoreactivity in the midbrain of adult rats: Regional, subregional, and cellular localization in the A10, A9, and A8 dopamine cell groups." *The Journal of Comparative Neurology.* (2002): 446, 288–300.

Daubner, S. C., T. Le, and S. Wang. "Tyrosine hydroxylase and Regulation of Dopamine Synthesis." *Archives of Biochemistry and Biophysics.* (2011 April 1): 508(1): 1–12.

David, V., L. Segu, M. C. Buhot, M. Ichaye, and P. Cazala. "Rewarding effects elicited by cocaine microinjections into the ventral tegmental area of C57BL/6 mice: Involvement of dopamine D(1) and serotonin(1B) receptors." *Psychopharmacology (Berl).* (2004): 174, 367–375.

De Dreu, C. K. "Oxytocin modulates cooperation within and competition between groups: An integrative review and research agenda." *Hormones and Behavior.* (2012): 57, 419–428.

Declerck, C. H., C. Boone, T. Kiyonari. "Oxytocin and cooperation under conditions of uncertainty: The modulating role of incentives and social information." *Hormones and Behavior.* (2010): 57, 368–374.

Den Hertog, C., A. de Groot, P. van Dongen. "History and use of oxytocics." *European Journal of Obstetrics and Gynecological and Reproductive Biology.* (2001): 94, 8–12.

Ditzen, B, M. Schaer, B. Gabriel, G. Bodenmann, U. Ehlert, M. Heinrichs. "Intranasal oxytocin increases positive communication and reduces cortisol levels during couple conflict." *Biological Psychiatry.* (2009): 65, 728–731.

Dluzen, D. E., V. D. Ramirez, C. S. Carter, L. L. Getz. "Male vole urine changes luteinizing hormone-releasing hormone and norepinephrine in female olfactory bulb." *Science.* (1981): 212, 573–575.

Donaldson, Z. R., L. Spiegel, L. J. Young. "Central vasopressin V1a receptor activation is independently necessary for both partner preference formation and expression in socially monogamous male prairie voles." *Behavioral Neuroscience.* (2010): 124, 159–163.

Donaldson, Z. R., L. J. Young. "Oxytocin, vasopressin, and the neurogenetics of sociality." *Science.* (2008): 322, 900–904.

Du Vigneaud, V. "Trail of sulfur research: From insulin to oxytocin." *Science.* (1956): 123, 967–74.

Ebstein, R. P., A. Knafo, D. Mankuta, S. H. Chew, P. S. Lai. "The contributions of oxytocin and vasopressin pathway genes to human behavior." *Hormones and Behavior.* (March, 2012):61(3): 359–79.

Eklunda, Anders, Thomas E. Nichols, and Hans Knutsson, "Cluster failure: Why fMRI inferences for spatial extent have inflated false-positive rates." *PNAS USA.* http://www.pnas.org/content/early/2016/06/27/1602413113.full.

Emanuele, E., M. Bertona, P. Minoretti, D. Geroldi. "An open-label trial of L-5-hydroxytryptophan in subjects with romantic stress." *Neuro Endocrinology Letters.* (2010): 31, 663–666.

Esposito, R. U., L. J. Porrino, T. F. Seeger, A. M. Crane, H. D. Everist, and A. Pert. "Changes in local cerebral glucose utilization during rewarding brain stimulation." *Proceedings of the National Academy of Sciences, USA.* (1984): 81, 635–639.

Etgen, A., J. C. Morales. "Somatosensory stimuli evoke norepinephrine release in the anterior ventromedial hypothalamus of sexually receptive female rats." *Journal of Neuroendocrinology.* (2002): 14, 213–218.

Etgen, A. M., H. P. Chu, J. M. Fiber, G. B. Karkanias, J. M. Morales. "Hormonal integration of neurochemical and sensory signals governing female reproductive behavior." *Behavioral Brain Research.* (1999):105, 93–103.

Evans, D. W., M. D. Lewis, E. Iobst. "The role of the orbitofrontal cortex in normally developing compulsive-like behaviors and obsessive-compulsive disorder." *Brain and Cognition.* (2004): 55, 220–234.

Fabre-Nys, C. "Male faces and odors evoke differential patterns of neurochemical release in the mediobasal hypothalamus of the ewe during estrus: An insight into sexual motivation." *European Journal of Neuroscience.* (1997): 9, 1666–1677.

Fabre-Nys, C. "Steroid control of monoamines in relation to sexual behaviour." *Reviews of Reproduction.* (1998): 3, 31–41.

Fair, D. A., A. L. Cohen, N. U. F. Dosenbach, J. A. Church, F. M. Miezin, D. M. Barch, M. E. Raichle, S. E. Petersen, B. L. Schlaggar. "The maturing architecture of the brain's default network." *The National Academy of Science of the USA.* (2008): 105(10): 4028–32. www.pnas.org/cgi/doi/10.1073/pnas.0800376105.

Feldman, R. "Oxytocin and social affiliation in humans." *Hormones and Behavior.* (2012): 61(3):380–391.

Feldman, R. "The relational basis of adolescent adjustment: Trajectories of mother-child interactive behaviors from infancy to adolescence shape adolescents' adaptation." *Attachment & Human Development.* (2010): 12, 173–192.

Feldman, R., A. Weller, J. F. Leckman, J. Kuint, A. I. Eidelman. "The nature of the mother's tie to her infant: Maternal bonding under conditions of proximity, separation, and potential loss." *Journal of Child Psychology and Psychiatry.* (1990): 40, 929–939.

Feldman, R., A. Weller, O. Zagoory-Sharon, A. Levine. "Evidence for a neuroendocrinological foundation of human affiliation: Plasma oxytocin levels across pregnancy and the postpartum period predict mother-infant bonding." *Psychological Science.* (2007): 18, 965–970.

Feldman, R., I. Gordon, I. Schneiderman, O. Weisman, O. Zagoory-Sharon. "Natural variations in maternal and paternal care are associated with systematic changes in oxytocin following parent-infant contact." *Psychoneuroendocrinology.* (2010): 35, 1133–1141.

Feldman, R., I. Gordon, O. Zagoory-Sharon. "Maternal and paternal plasma, salivary, and urinary oxytocin and parent-infant synchrony: Considering stress and affiliation components of human bonding." *Developmental Science.* (2011): 14, 752–761.

Feldman, R., P. S. Klein. "Toddlers' self-regulated compliance to mothers, caregivers, and fathers: Implications for theories of socialization." *Developmental Psychology.* (2003): 39, 680–692.

Feldman, R., S. Masalha. "Parent-child and triadic antecedents of children's social competence: cultural specificity, shared process." *Developmental Psychology.* (2010): 46, 455–467.

Ferrari, F., D. Giuliani. "Sexual attraction and copulation in male rats: Effects of the dopamine agonist SND 919." *Pharmacology, Biochemistry, and Behavior.* (1995): 50, 29–34.

Fiorino, D. F, A. Coury, A. G. Phillips. "Dynamic changes in nucleus accumbens dopamine efflux during the Coolidge effect in male rats." *Journal of Neuroscience.* (1997):17, 4849–4855.

Fisher, H., PhD. *The Anatomy of Love: A Natural History of Mating, Marriage, and Why We Stray.* New York: W. W. Norton & Company. (2016). ISBN-13: 978-0393349740.

Forsling, M. L., H. Montgomery, D. Halpin, R. J. Windle, D. F. Treacher. "Daily patterns of secretion of neurohypophysial hormones in man: Effect of age." *Experimental Physiology.* (1998): 83, 409–418.

Freeman, S. M., H. Walum, K. Inoue, A. L. Smith, M. M. Goodman, K. L. Bales, L. J. Young. "Neuroanatomical distribution of oxytocin and vasopressin 1a receptors in the socially monogamous coppery titi monkey (Callicebus cupreus)." *Neuroscience*. (July 25, 2014): 273: 12–23.

Fuchs, A. R., O. Behrens, H. C. Lin. "Correlation of nocturnal increase in plasma oxytocin in plasma with a decrease in estadiol/progesterone ratio in late pregnancy." *American Journal of Obstetrics and Gynecology*. (1992): 167, 1559–63.

Furman, D. J., M. C. Chen, I. A. Gotlib. "Variant in oxytocin receptor gene is associated with amygdala volume." *Psychoneuroendocrinology*. (July, 2011): 36(6): 891–97.

Galfi, M. T. Janaky, R. Toth, G. Prohaszka, C. Juhasz, C. Varga, and F. A. Laszlo. "Effects of dopamine and dopamine-active compounds on oxytocin and vasopressin production in rat neurohypophyseal tissue cultures." *Regulatory Peptides*. (2001): 98, 49–54.

Garver-Apgar, C. E., S. W. Gangestad, R. Thornhill, R. D. Millare, and J. J. Olp. "Major histocompatibility complex alleles, sexual responsivity, and unfaithfulness in romantic couples." *Psychological Science*. (October, 2006): 17(10): 830–5.

Gavrilets, S. "Human origins and the transition from promiscuity to pair-bonding." *Proceedings of the National Academy of Sciences, USA*. (2012): 109(25): 9923–9928.

Gerfen, C. R, M. Herkenham, and J. Thibault. "The neostriatal mosaic: II. Patch- and matrix-directed mesostriatal dopaminergic and non-dopaminergic systems." *Journal of Neuroscience*. (1987): 7, 3915–3934.

Gimpl, G., and F. Fahrenholz. "The oxytocin receptor system: Structure, function, and regulation." *Physiological Reviews*. (2001): 81, 629–83.

Gingrich., B, Y. Liu, C. Z. Cascio, and T. R. Insel. "Dopamine D2 receptors in the nucleus accumbens are important for social attachment in female prairie voles (Microtus ochrogaster)." *Behavioral Neuroscience*. (2000): 114, 173–183.

Ginsberg, S. D., P. R. Hof, W. G. Young, and J. H. Morrison. "Noradrenergic innervation of vasopressin- and oxytocin-containing neurons in the hypothalamic paraventricular nucleus of the macaque monkey: Quantitative analysis using double-label immunohistochemistry and confocal laser microscopy." *The Journal of Comparative Neurology*. (1994): 341, 476–491.

Gonzaga, G. C., R. A. Turner, D. Keltner, B. Campos, and M. Altemus. "Romantic love and sexual desire in close relationships." *Emotion*. (2006): 6, 163–179.

Gordon, I., C. Martin, R. Feldman, and J. F. Leckman. "Oxytocin and social motivation." *Developmental Cognitive Neuroscience*. (2011): 1, 471–493.

Gordon, I., O. Zagoory-Sharon, J. F. Leckman, R. Feldman. "Oxytocin and the development of parenting in humans." *Biological Psychiatry*. (2010): 68, 377–382.

Gordon, I., O. Zagoory-Sharon, J. F. Leckman, and R. Feldman. "Oxytocin, cortisol, and triadic family interactions." *Physiology and Behavior*. (2010): 101, 679–684.

Gordon, I., O. Zagoory-Sharon, I. Schneiderman, J. F. Leckman, A. Weller, and R. Feldman. "Oxytocin and cortisol in romantically unattached young adults: Associations with bonding and psychological distress." *Psychophysiology.* (2008): 45, 349–352.

Green, C. G., et al. "Prenatal maternal depression and child serotonin transporter linked polymorphic region (5-HTTLPR) and dopamine receptor D4 (DRD4) genotype predict negative emotionality from 3 to 36 months." *Developmental Psychopathology.* (July 18, 2016): 1–17.

Grewen, K. M., S. S. Girdler, J. Amico, and K. C. Light. "Effects of partner support on resting oxytocin, cortisol, norepinephrine, and blood pressure before and after warm partner contact." *Psychosomatic Medicine.* (2005): 67(4): 531–538.

Griffin, M. G., and G. T. Taylor. "Norepinephrine modulation of social memory: Evidence for a time-dependent functional recovery of behavior." *Behavioral Neuroscience.* (1995): 109, 466–473.

Guastella, A. J., P. B. Mitchell, and M. R. Dadds. "Oxytocin increases gaze to the eye region of human faces." *Biological Psychiatry.* (2008): 63, 3–5.

Guiard, B. P., M. El Mansari, and P. Blier. "Cross-talk between dopaminergic and noradrenergic systems in the rat ventral tegmental area, locus ceruleus and dorsal hippocampus." *Molecular Pharmacology.* (November, 2008):74(5): 1463–75.

Guiard, B. P., M. El Mansari, and P. Blier. "Prospect of a dopamine contribution in the next generation of antidepressant drugs; the triple reuptake inhibitors." *Current Drug Targets.* (November, 2009):10(11): 1069 –84.

Guiard B. P., M. El Mansari, Z. Merali, and P. Blier. "Functional interactions between dopamine, serotonin and norepinephrine neurons: An in vivo electrophysiological study in rats with monoaminogenic leasions." *International Journal of Neuropharmacology.* (August, 2008):11(5): 625–39.

Gunst, A., et al. "A study of possible associations between single nucleotide polymorphisms in the estrogen receptor 2 gene and female sexual desire." *The Journal of Sexual Medicine.* (March, 2015):12(3): 676–84.

Gupta, J., R. Russell, C. Wayman, D. Hurley, and V. Jackson. "Oxytocin-induced contractions within rat and rabbit ejaculatory tissues are mediated by vasopressin V1A receptors and not oxytocin receptors." *British Journal of Pharmacology.* (2008): 155, 118–26.

Hammock, E. A. D., and L. J. Young. "Microsatellite instability generates diversity in brain and sociobehavioral traits." *Science.* (2005): 308, 1630–1634.

Harris, C. R., and N. Christenfeld. "Gender, jealousy, and reason." *Psychological Science.* (1996): 7, 364–366.

Hatfield, E., and S. Sprecher. "Measuring passionate love in intimate relationships." *Journal of Adolescence.* (1986): 9, 383–410.

Hatfield E., E. Schmitz, J. Cornelius, and R. L. Rapson. "Passionate love: How early does it begin?" *Journal of Psychology and Human Sexuality.* (1988): 1: 35–51.

Hayduk, L. A. "Personal space: where we now stand." *Psychological Bulletin.* (1983): 94, 293–335.

Hazan, C., and L. M. Diamond. "The place of attachment in human mating." *Review of General Psychology.* (2000): 4, 186–204.

Hazan, C., and P. R. Shaver. "Romantic love conceptualized as an attachment process." *Journal of Personal and Social Psychology.* (1987): 52, 511–524.

Heon-Jin, L., A. H. Macbeth, J. Pagani and W. C. Young. "Oxytocin: The great facilitator of life." *Progress in Neurobiology.* (June, 2009): 88(2): 127–151.

Herbert, J. "Sexuality, stress and the chemical architecture of the brain." *Annual Review of Sexual Research.* (1996): 7, 1–44.

Hollander, E., S. Novotny, M. Hanratty, R. Yaffe, C. M. DeCaria, and B. R. Aronowitz, et al. "Oxytocin infusion reduces repetitive behaviors in adults with autistic and Asperger's disorders." *Neuropsychopharmacology.* (2003): 28, 193–8.

Hollerman, J. R., L. Tremblay, and W. Schultz. "Involvement of basal ganglia and orbitofrontal cortex in goal-directed behavior." *Progress in Brain Research.* (2000): 126, 193–215.

Holt-Lunstad, J., W. A. Birmingham, and K. C. Light. "Influence of a 'warm touch' support enhancement intervention among married couples on ambulatory blood pressure, oxytocin, alpha amylase, and cortisol." *Psychosomatic Medicine.* (2008): 70, 976–985.

Horvitz, J. C., T. Stewart, and B. L. Jacobs. "Burst activity of ventral tegmental dopamine neurons is elicited by sensory stimuli in the awake cat." *Brain Research.* (1997): 759, 251–258.

Howell, W. H. "The physiological effects of extracts of the hypophysis cerebri and infundibular body." *The Journal of Experimental Medicine.* (1989): 3, 245–58.

Hrynaszkiewicz, I. *Nature.com.* Blog post, July 2016. "Promoting research data sharing at Springer Nature." http://blogs.nature.com/ofschemesand memes/2016/07/05/promoting-research-data-sharing-at-springer-nature.

Hull, E. M., J. Du, D. S. Lorrain, and L. Matuszewich. "Extracellular dopamine in the medial preoptic area: Implications for sexual motivation and hormonal control of copulation." *The Journal of Neuroscience.* (1995): 15, 7465–7471.

Hull, E. M., J. Du, D. S. Lorrain, and L. Matuszewick. "Testosterone, preoptic dopamine, and copulation in male rats." *Brain Research Bulletin.* (1997): 44, 327–333.

Hull, E. M., D. S. Lorrain, J. Du, L. Matuszewick, L. A. Lumley, S. K. Putnam, and J. Moses. "Hormone-neurotransmitter interactions in the control of sexual behavior." *Behavioral Brain Research.* (1996): 105, 105–116.

Hurlemann, R., A. Patin, O. A. Onur, M. X. Cohen, T. Baumgartner, S. Metzler, I. Dziobek, J. Gallinat, M. Wagner, K. Maier, and K. M. Kendrick. "Oxytocin enhances amygdala-dependent, socially reinforced learning and emotional empathy in humans." *The Journal of Neuroscience.* (2010): 30, 4999–5007.

Insel, T. R., and T. J. Hulihan. "A gender-specific mechanism for pair-bonding: oxytocin and partner preference formation in monogamous voles." *Behavioral Neuroscience.* (1995): 109, 782–789.

Insel, T. R., L. Young, and Z. Wang. "Molecular aspects of monogamy." *Annals of the New York Academy of Sciences.* (1997): 807, 302–316.

Insel, T. R. "The challenge of translation in social neuroscience: A review of oxytocin, vasopressin, and affiliative behavior." *Neuron.* (2010): 65(6): 768–779.

Israel, S., et al. "Molecular genetic studies of the arginine vasopressin 1a receptor (AVPR1a) in human behavior: from autism to altruism with some notes in between." *Progress in Brain Research.* (2008): 170: 435–49.

Jaffee, D. J., *Huffington Post,* 8/6/2013, "Review: *Brainwashed: The seductive appeal of mindless neuroscience.*" http://www.huffingtonpost.com/dj-jaffe/brain washed-the-seductive_b_3712860.html.

Jankowiak, W. R., and E. F. Fischer. "A cross-cultural perspective on romantic love." *Ethnology.* (1992): 31, 149–155.

Jin, D., H. X. Liu, H. Hirai, T. Torashima, T. Nagai, O. Lopatina, N. A. Shnayder, K. Yamada, M. Noda, T. Seike, K. Fujita, S. Takasawa, S. Yokoyama, K. Koizumi, Y. Shiraishi, S. Tanaka, M. Hashii, T. Yoshihara, K. Higashida, M. S. Islam, N. Yamada, K. Hayashi, N. Noguchi, I. Kato, H. Okamoto, A. Matsushima, A. Salmina, T. Munesue, N. Shimizu, S. Mochida, M. Asano, and H. Higashida. "CD38 is critical for social behavior by regulating oxytocin secretion." *Nature.* (2007): 446, 41–45.

Kagerer, S., T. Klucken, S. Wehrum, M. Zimmermann, A. Schienle, B. Walter, D. Vaitl, and R. Stark. "Neural activation toward erotic stimuli in homosexual and heterosexual males." *The Journal of Sexual Medicine.* (November, 2011): 8(11): 3132–43.

Kalivas, P. W., and P. Duffy. "Repeated cocaine administration alters extracellular glutamate in the ventral tegmental area." *Journal of Neurochemistry.* (1998): 70: 1497–1502.

Kampe, K. K., C. D. Frith, R. J. Dolan, and U. Frith. "Reward value of attractiveness and gaze." *Nature.* (2001): 413, 589.

Kavaliers, M., E. Choleris, A. Agmo, W. J. Braun, D. D. Colwell, and L. J. Muglia, et al. "Inadvertent social information and the avoidance of parasitized male mice: A role for oxytocin." *Proceedings of the National Academy of Sciences, USA.* (2006): 103, 4293–8.

Kawagoe, R., Y. Takikawa, and O. Hikosaka. "Expectation of reward modulates cognitive signals in the basal ganglia." *Nature Neuroscience.* (1998): 1, 411–416.

Kawashima, S., K. Takagi. "Role of sex steroids on the survival, neuritic outgrowth of neurons, and dopamine neurons in cultured preoptic area and hypothalamus." *Hormones and Behavior.* (1994): 28, 305–312.

Keath, J. R., et al. "Differential Modulation by Nicotine of Substantia Nigra versus Ventral Tegmental Area Dopamine Neurons." *Journal of Neurophysiology.* (December, 2007): 98(6):3388–96.

Kemp, Ah, and A. J. Guastella. "The role of oxytocin in human affect: a novel hypothesis." *Current Directions in Psychological Science.* (2011): 20, 222–231.

Kemp, J. M., and T. P. Powell. "The cortico-striate projection in the monkey." *Brain.* (1970): 93, 525–546.

Kendrick, K. M, and A. F. Dixson. "Anteromedial hypothalamic lesions block proceptivity but not receptivity in the female common marmoset (Callithrix jacchus)." *Brain Research.* (1986): 375, 221–229.

Kendrick, K. M., E. B. Keverne, M. R. Hinton, and J. A. Goode. "Oxytocin, amino acid and monoamine release in the region of the medial preoptic area and bed nucleus of the stria terminalis of the sheep during parturition and suckling." *Brain Research.* (1992): 569, 199–209.

Kendrick, K. M. "Oxytocin, motherhood and bonding." *Experimental Physiology.* (2000): 85S, 111S–124S.

Kendrick, K. M. "The neurobiology of social bonds." *Journal of Neuroendocrinology.* (2004): 16, 1007–8.

Kennedy, D. P., J. Glascher, J. M. Tyszkaa, and R. Adolphs. "Personal space regulation by the human amygdalla." *Nature Neuroscience.* (2009): 12, 1226–1227.

Kleiman, D. G. "Monogamy in mammals." *The Quarterly Review of Biology.* (1997): 52: (1): 39–69.

Kohtz, A. S., and G. Aston-Jones. "Cocaine Seeking during Initial Abstinence is Driven by Noradrenergic and Serotonergic Signaling in Hippocampus in Sex-Dependent Manner." *Neuropsychopharmacology.* (2016): Sep 14.

Kosfeld, M., M. Heinrichs, P. Zak, U. Fischbacher, and E. Fehr. "Oxytocin increases trust in humans." *Nature.* (2005): 435, 673–6.

Kovacs, G., and G. Telegdy. "Effects of oxytocin, des-glycinamide-oxytocin and anti-oxytocin serum on the alpha-MPT-induced disappearance of catecholamines in the rat brain." *Brain Research.* (1983): 268, 307–314.

Kovacs, G. L., Z. Sarnyai, E. Barbarczi, G. Szabo, and G. Telegdy. "The role of oxytocin-dopamine interactions in cocaine-induced locomotor hyperactivity." *Neuropharmacology.* (1990): 29, 365–368.

Kovacs, G. L., Z. Sarnyai, and G. Szabo. "Oxytocin and addiction: A review." *Psychoneuroendocrinology.* (1998): 23, 945–62.

Koyama, S., M. S. Brodie, S. B. Appel. "Ethanol Inhibition of M-current and Ethanol-Induced Direct Excitation of Ventral Tegmental Area Dopamine Neurons." *Journal of Neurophysiology.* (March, 2007): 97(3):1977–85.

Kramer, Samuel Noah. *History Begins at Sumer.* Philadelphia: University of Pennsylvania Press. (1956). ISBN: 0-8122-1276-2.

Kruger, T. H., P. Haake, D. Chereath, W. Knapp, O. E. Janssen, M. S. Exton, M. Schedlowski, and J. I. Hartmann. "Specificity of the neuroendocine response to orgasm during sexual arousal in men." *The Journal of Endocrinology.* (2003): 177, 57–64.

Kumsta, R., and M. Heinrichs. "Oxytocin, stress and social behavior: neurogenetics of the human oxytocin system." *Current Opinion in Neurobiology.* (February, 2013): 23(1): 11–6.

Lauwereyns, J., Y. Takikawa, R. Kawagoe, S. Kobayashi, M. Koizumi, B. Coe, M. Sakagami, and O. Hikosaka. "Feature-based anticipation of cues that predict reward in monkey caudate nucleus." *Neuron.* (2002): 33, 463–473.

Lavin, A., L. Nogueira, C. C. Lapish, R. M. Wightman, P. E. M. Phillips, and J. K. Seamans. "Mesocortical dopamine neurons operate in distinct temporal domains using multimodal signaling." *The Journal of Neuroscience.* (2005): 25, 5013–5023.

Legault, M., and R. A. Wise. "Injections of N-methyl-d-asparate into the ventral hippocampus increase extracellular dopamine in the ventral tegmental area and nucleus accumbens." *Synapse.* (1999): 31, 241–249.

Legros, J. J. "Inhibitory effect of oxytocin on corticotrope function in humans: Are vasopressin and oxytocin ying-yang neurohormones?" *Psychoneuroendocrinology.* (2001): 26, 649–55.

Levine, A., O. Zagoory-Sharon, R. Feldman, and A. Weller. "Oxytocin during pregnancy and early postpartum: individual patterns and maternal-fetal attachment." *Peptides.* (2007): 28, 1162–1169.

Lian, J., B. Pan, and C. Deng. "Early antipsychotic exposure affects serotonin and dopamine receptor binding density differently in selected brain loci of male and female juvenile rats." *Pharmacological Reports.* (July, 2016): 15:68(5): 1028–1035.

Light, K. C., K. M. Grewen, and J. A. Amico. "More frequent partner hugs and higher oxytocin levels are linked to lower blood pressure and heart rate in premenopausal women." *Biological Psychology.* (2005): 69(1): 5–21.

Lim, M. M., A. Z. Murphy, and A. J. Young. "Ventral striatopallidal oxytocin and vasopressin V1a receptors in the monogamous prairie vole (Microtus ochrogaster)." *The Journal of Comparative Neurology.* (2004): 468, 555–570.

Lim, M. M, Z. Wang, D. E. Olazabal, X. Ren, E. F. Terwilliger, and L. J. Young. "Enhanced partner preference in a promiscuous species by manipulating the expression of a single gene." *Nature.* (2004): 429, 754–757.

Lim, M. M, and L. J. Young. "Vasopressin-dependent neural circuits underlying pair bond formation in the monogamous prairie vole." *Neuroscience.* (2004): 125(1): 35–45.

Liu, J., P. Gong, and X. Zhou. "The association between romantic relationship status and 5-HT1A gene in young adults." *Scientific Reports.* (2014): 4: 7049.

Liu, Y., and Z. X. Wang. "Nucleus accumbens oxytocin and dopamine interact to regulate pair bond formation in female prairie voles." *Neuroscience.* (2003): 121, 537–544.

Liu, Y., J. T. Curtis, and Z. Wang. "Vasopressin in the lateral septum regulates pair bond formation in male prairie voles (Microtus ochrogaster)." *Behavioral Neuroscience.* (2001): 115, 910–919.

Liu, Y., Z. X. Wang. "Nucleus accumbens oxytocin and dopamine interact to regulate pair bond formation in female prairie voles." *Neuroscience.* (2003): 121(3): 537–544.

Liu, Y. C., B. D. Sachs, and J. D. Salamone. "Sexual behavior in male rats after radiofrequency or dopamine-depleting lesions in nucleus accumbens." *Pharmacology, Biochemistry, and Behavior.* (1998): 60, 585–592.

Logothetis, N. K., J. Pauls, M. Augath, T. Trinath, and A. Oeltermann. "Neurophysiological investigation of the basis of the fMRI signal." *Nature.* (2001): 412, 150–157.

Love, T. "Oxytocin, Motivation and the role of Dopamine." *Pharmacology, Biochemistry, and Behavior.* (April, 2014): 0: 49–60.

Love, T. M., et al. "Oxytocin gene polymorphisms influence human dopaminergic function in a sex-dependent manner." *Biological Psychiatry.* (2012): 72(3): 198–206.

Luijkx, T., and A. Prof F. Gaillard, et al. Radiopaedia.org. Radiologist's opinion of fMRI. http://radiopaedia.org/articles/functional-mri.

Luo, S., D. Yu, and S. Han. "Genetic and neural correlates of romantic relationship satisfaction." *Social Cognitive and Affective Neuroscience.* (February, 2016): 11(2): 337–48.

Magon, N., and S. Kalra. "The orgasmic history of oxytocin: Love, lust and labor." *Indian Journal of Endocrinology and Metabolism.* (September, 2011): 15(Suppl3): S156–S161.

Mahovetz, L. M., L. J. Young, and W. D. Hopkins. "The influence of AVPR1A Genotype on Individual Differences in Behaviors During a Mirror Self-Recognition Task in Chimpanzees (Pan troglodytes)." *Genes, Brain, and Behavior.* (2016): Apr 5.

Manning, M., S. Stoev, B. Chini, T. Durroux, B. Mouillac, and G. Guillon. "Peptide and non-peptide agonists and antagonists for the vasopressin and oxytocin V1a, V1b, V2 and OT receptors: Research tools and potential therapeutic agents." *Progress in Brain Research.* (2008): 170, 473–512.

Marazziti, D., H. S. Akiskal, A. Rossi, and G. B. Cassano. "Alteration of the platelet serotonin transporter in romantic love." *Psychological Medicine.* (1999): 29, 741–745.

Marazziti, D., D. and D. Canale. "Hormonal changes when falling in love." *Psychoneuroendocrinology.* (2004): 29, 931–936.

Marazziti, D., B. Dell'Osso, S. Baroni, F. Mungai, M. Catena, P. Rucci, F. Albanese, G. Giannaccini, L. Betti, L. Fabbrini, P. Italiani, A. Del Debbio, A. Lucacchini, and L. Dell'Osso. "A relationship between oxytocin and anxiety of romantic attachment." *Clinical Practice and Epidemiology in Mental Health.* (2006): 2, 28.

Marazziti, D., I. Roncaglia, A. Del Debbio, C. Bianchi, G. Massimetti, N. Origlia, L. Domenici, A. Piccinni, L. Dell'Osso. "Brain-derived neurotrophic factor in romantic attachment." *Psychological Medicine.* (2009): 39, 1927–1930.

Margolis, E. B., et al. "Both Kappa and Mu opioid Agonists Inhibit Glutamatergic Input to Ventral Tegmental Area Neurons." *Journal of Neurophysiology.* (June, 2005): 93(6): 3086–93.

Martin-Soelch, C., K. L. Leenders, A. F. Chevalley, J. Missimer, G. Kunig, S. Magyar, A. Mino, and W. Schultz. "Reward mechanisms in the brain and their role in dependence: Evidence from neurophysiological and neuroimaging studies." *Brain Research Reviews.* (2001): 36, 139–149.

Masarik, A. S., R. D. Conger, M. B. Donnellan, M. C. Stallings, M. J. Martin, T. J. Schofield, T. K. Neppl, L. V. Scaramella, A. Smolen, and K. F. Widaman. "For better and for worse: genes and parenting interact to predict future behavior in romantic relationships." *Journal of Family Psychology.* (June, 2014): 28(3): 357–67.

Matsunaga, M., S. Sato, T. Isowa, H. Tsuboi, T. Konagaya, H. Kaneko, and H. Ohira. "Profiling of serum proteins influenced by warm partner contact in healthy couples." *Neuro Endocrinology Letters.* (2009): 30, 227–236.

Mattick, R. P., and J. C. Clarke. "Development and validation measures of social phobia scrutiny fear and social interaction anxiety." *Behavioral Research and Therapy.* (1998): 36, 455–470.

McBride, W. J., J. M. Murphy, and S. Ikemoto. "Localization of brain reinforcement mechanisms: Intracranial self-administration and intracranial place-conditioning studies." *Behavioral Brain Research.* (1999): 101, 129–152.

McCall, C., and T. Singer. "The animal and human neuroendocrinology of social cognition, motivation, and behavior." *Nature Neuroscience.* (2012): 15, 681–688.

Meiser, J., et al. "Complexity of dopamine metabolism." *Cell Communication and Signaling.* (2013): 11:34.

Melse, M., Y. Temel, S. K. Tan, and A. Jahanshahi. "Deep brain stimulation of the rostromedial tegmental nucleus: An unanticipated, selective effect on food intake." *Brain Research Bulletin.* (August 9, 2016): 127: 23–28.

Mever-Lindenberg, A., G. Domes, P. Kirsch, and M. Heinrichs. "Oxytocin and vasopressin in the human brain: social neuropeptides for translational medicine." *Nature Reviews Neuroscience.* (2011): 12, 524–538.

Miller, Greg. *Science.* "Brain scans are prone to false positives, study says." (July 2016) http://www.sciencemagazinedigital.org/sciencemagazine/15_ july_2016_Main?sub_id=UI36dy9C7O4Y&u1=41481570&folio=232&pg=16 #pg16.

Moles, A., B. L. Kieffer, and F. R. D'Amato. "Deficit in attachment behavior in mice lacking the u-opioid receptor gene." *Science.* (2004): 304, 1983–1985.

Montague, P. R., S. M. McClure, R. P. Baldwin, P. E. Phillips, E. A. Budygin, G. D. Stuber, M. R. Kilpatrick, and R. M. Wightman. "Dynamic gain control of dopamine delivery in freely moving animals." *The Journal of Neuroscience.* (2004): 24, 1754–1759.

Montejo, A. L., L. Montejo, and F. Navarro-Cremades. "Sexual side-effects of anti-depressant and antipsychotic drugs." *Current Opinion in Psychiatry*. (November, 2015): 28(6): 418–23.

Morcom, A. M., and P. C. Fletcher. "Does the brain have a baseline? Why we should be resisting a rest." *NeuroImage*. (2007): 37: 1073–1082.

Morhenn, V., L. E. Beavin, and P. J. Zak. "Massage increases oxytocin and reduces adrenocorticotropin hormone in humans." *Alternative Therapies in Health and Medicine*. (2012): 18(6):11–18.

Murray, S. L., et al. "Tempting fate or inviting happiness? Unrealistic idealization prevents the decline of marital satisfaction." *Psychological Science*. (2011): 22(5):619–626.

Neff, B. D., and T. E. Pitcher. "Genetic quality and sexual selection: An integrated framework for good genes and compatible genes." *Molecular Ecology*. (January, 2005): 14(1): 19–38.

Neumann, I. D. "The advantage of social living: Brain neuropeptides mediate the beneficial consequences of sex and motherhood." *Frontiers in Neuroendocrinology*. (2009): 30, 483–96.

Nickerson, K., R. W. Bonsness, R. G. Douglas, P. Condliffe, and V. du Vigneaud. "Oxytocin and milk ejection." *American Journal of Obstetrics and Gynecology*. (1954): 67, 1028–34.

O'Doherty, J., P. Dayan, J. Schultz, R. Deichmann, K. Friston, and R. J. Dolan. "Dissociable roles of ventral and dorsal striatum in instrumental conditioning." *Science*. (2004): 304, 452–454.

Oades, R. D., and G. M. Halliday. "Ventral tegmental (A10) system: neurobiology. 1. Anatomy and connectivity." *Brain Research*. (1987): 434, 117–165.

Okun, M. S., J. Green, R. Saben, R. Gross, K. D. Foote, and J. L. Vitek. "Mood changes with deep brain stimulation of STN and Gpi: Results of a pilot study." *Journal of Neurology, Neurosurgery, and Psychiatry*. (2003): 74: 1584–1586.

Olds, J., and P. Milner. "Positive reinforcement produced by electrical stimulation of septal area and other regions of rat brain." *Journal of Comparative and Physiological Psychology*. (1954): 47, 419–427.

Oliver, G., and E. A. Schäfer. "On the physiological action of extracts of pituitary body and certain other glandular organs: Preliminary communication." *The Journal of Physiology*. (1895): 18, 277–9.

Ophir, A. G., A. Gessel, D. J. Zheng, and S. M. Phelps. "Oxytocin receptor density is associated with male mating tactics and social monogamy." *Hormones and Behavior*. (2012): 61(3): 445–453.

Parent, A., and L. N. Hazrati. "Functional anatomy of the basal ganglia. I. The cortico-basal ganglia-thalamo-cortical loop." *Brain Research. Brain Research Reviews*. (1995): 20, 91–127.

Paul, Thomas, B. Schiffer, T. Zwarg, T. H. Krüger, S. Karama, M. Schedlowski, M. Forsting, and E. R. Gizewski. "Brain response to visual sexual stimuli in heterosexual and homosexual males." *Human Brain Mapping*. (June, 2008): 29(6): 726–35.

Peabody, Susan. *Addiction to Love: Overcoming obsession and dependency in relationships*. Berkeley: Celestial Arts. (2005). ISBN-13: 978-0890877159.

Pfaff, D., J. Frohlich, and M. Morgan. "Hormonal and genetic influences on arousal—sexual and otherwise." *Trends in Neurosciences*. (2002): 25, 45–50.

Phillips, P. E., G. D. Stuber, M. L. Heien, R. M. Wightman, and R. M. Carelli. "Subsecond dopamine release promotes cocaine seeking." *Nature*. (2003): 422, 614–618.

Pierce, J. G., and V. du Vigneaud. "Studies on high potency oxytocic material from beef posterior pituitary lobes." *The Journal of Biological Chemistry*. (1950): 186, 77–84.

Pitkow, L. J., C. A. Sharer, C. X. Ren, T. R. Insel, E. F. Terwilliger, and L. J. Young. "Facilitation of affiliation and pair-bond formation by vasopressin receptor gene transfer into the ventral forebrain of a monogamous vole." *The Journal of Neuroscience*. (2001): 21, 7392–7396.

Porrino, L. J., R. U. Esposito, T. F. Seeger, A. M. Crane, A. Pert, and L. Sokoloff. "Metabolic mapping of the brain during rewarding self-stimulation." *Science*. (1984): 224, 306–309.

Porrino, L. J., D. Huston-Lyons, G. Bain, L. Sokoloff, and C. Kornetsky. "The distribution of changes in local cerebral energy metabolism associated with brain stimulation reward to the medial forebrain bundle of the rat." *Brain Research*. (1990): 511, 1–6.

Posner, M., and S. Petersen. "The attention system of the human brain." *Annual Review of Neuroscience*. (1990): 13, 25–42.

Redoute, J., S. Stoleru, M. C. Gregoire, N. Costes, L. Cinotti, F. Lavenne, D. Le Bars, M. G. Forest, and J. F. Pujol. "Brain processing of visual sexual stimuli in human males." *Human Brain Mapping*. (2000): 11, 162–177.

Resource. Free fMRI software. http://www.fil.ion.ucl.ac.uk/spm.

Resource. PubMed. http://www.ncbi.nlm.nih.gov/pubmed.

Resource. WikiDoc. http://www.wikidoc.org/index.php/Main_Page.

Resource. Wikipedia. https://en.wikipedia.org

Rice, M. E., S. J. Cragg, and S. A. Greenfield. "Characteristics of Electrically Evoked Somatodendritic Dopamine Release in Substantia Nigra and Ventral Tegmental Area In Vitro." *Journal of Neurophysiology*. (February, 1997): Vol. 77 no. 2, 853–862.

Ridderinkhof, K. R., W. P. van den Wildenberg, S. J. Segalowitz, and C. S. Carter. "Neurocognitive mechanisms of cognitive control: The role of prefrontal cortex in action selection, response inhibition, performance monitoring, and reward-based learning." *Brain and Cognition*. (2004): 56, 129–140.

Robbins, T., S. Granon, J. Muir, P. Durantou, A. Harrison, and B. Everitt. "Neural systems underlying arousal and attention: implications for drug abuse." *Annals of the New York Academy of Sciences*. (1998): 846, 222–237.

Robbins, T. W., and B. J. Everitt. "Neurobehavioural mechanisms of reward and motivation." *Current Opinion in Neurobiology.* (1996): 6, 228–236.

Robinson, D. L., M. L. Heien, and R. M. Wightman. "Frequency of dopamine concentration transients increases in dorsal and ventral striatum of male rats during introduction of conspecifics." *The Journal of Neuroscience.* (2002): 22, 10477–10486.

Romero-Fernandez, W., D. O. Borroto-Escuela, L. F. Agnati, and K. Fuxe. "Evidence for the existence of dopamine D2-oxytocin receptor heteromers in the ventral and dorsal striatum with faciliatory receptor-receptor interactions." *Molecular Psychiatry.* (2013): 18(8): 849–850.

Rosen, R. C., R. M. Lane, and M. Menza. "Effects of SSRIs on sexual function: a critical review." *Journal of Clinical Psychopharmacology.* (1999): 19, 67–85.

Ross, H. E., and L. J. Young. "Oxytocin and the neural mechanisms regulating social cognition and affiliative behavior." *Frontiers in Neuroendocrinology.* (2009): 30, 534–547.

Saint-Cyr, J. A., L. G. Ungerleider, and R. Desimone. "Organization of visual cortical inputs to the striatum and subsequent outputs to the pallido-nigral complex in the monkey." *The Journal of Comparative Neurology.* (1990): 298, 129–156.

Salinas, J. A., and N. M. White. "Contributions of the hippocampus, amygdala, and dorsal striatum to the response elicited by reward reduction." *Behavioral Neuroscience.* (1998): 112, 812–826.

Satel, S., MD. *Brainwashed: The seductive appeal of mindless neuroscience.* Basic Books: New York. (2015). ISBN-13: 978-0465062911.

Satel, S., MD. "Don't read too much into brain scans." *Time.* (May 30, 2013). http://ideas.time.com/2013/05/30/dont-read-too-much-into-brain-scans.

Schaschl, H., et al. "Signature of positive selection in the Cis-regulatory sequences of human oxytocin receptor (OXRT) and arginine vasopressin receptor 1a (AVPR1A) genes." *BMC Evolutionary Biology.* (2015): 15: 85.

Scheele, D., et al. "Oxytocin modulates social distance between males and females." *The Journal of Neuroscience.* (2012): 32(46): 16074–16079.

Scheele, D., A. Wille, K. Kendrick, B. Stoffel-Wagner, B. Becker, O. Gunturkun, W. Maier, and R. Hurlemann. "Oxytocin enhances brain reward system responses in men viewing the face of their female partner." *Proceedings of the National Academy of Sciences, USA.* (December 10, 2013): 110(50): 20308–20313.

Schiffler, P. T., et al. "Brain response to visual sexual stimuli in heterosexual and homosexual males." *Human Brain Mapping.* (June, 2008): 29(6): 726–35.

Schneiderman, I., Y. Kanat-Maymon, R. P. Ebstein, and R. Feldman. "Cumulative risk on the oxytocin receptor gene (OXTR) underpins empathic communication difficulties at first stages of romantic love." *Social Cognitive and Affective Neuroscience.* (October, 2014): 9(10): 1524–9.

Schneiderman, I., O. Zagoory-Sharon, J. F. Leckman, and R. Feldman. "Oxytocin during the initial stages of romantic attachment: Relations to couples' interactive reciprocity." *Psychoneuroendocrinology*. (2012): 37(8):1277–1285.

Schorscher-Pectu, A., S. Sotocinal, S. Ciura, A. Dupre, J. Ritchie, R. E. Sorge, J. N. Crawley, S. B. Hu, K. Nishimori, L. J. Young, F. Tribollet, R. Quirion, and J. S. Mogil. "Oxytocin-induced analgesia and scratching are mediated by the vasopressin-1A receptor in the mouse." *The Journal of Neuroscience*. (2010): 30, 8274–8284.

Schultz, W. "Multiple reward signals in the brain." *Nature Reviews. Neuroscience*. (2000): 1, 199–207.

Schwarzberg, H., G. L. Kovacs, G. Szabo, and G. Telegdy. "Intraventricular administration of vasopressin and oxytocin affects the steady-state levels of serotonin, dopamine and norepinephrine in rat brain." *Endocrinologia Experimentalis*. (1981): 15, 75–80.

Scicurious. "IgNobel Prize in Neuroscience: The dead salmon study." Blog post, September 25, 2012. http://blogs.scientificamerican.com/scicurious-brain/ ignobel-prize-in-neuroscience-the-dead-salmon-study.

Seagraves, R. T., H. Croft, R. Kavoussi, J. A. Ascher, S. R. Batey, V. J. Foster, C. Bolden-Watson, and A. Metz. "Bupropion sustained release (SR) for treatment of hypoactive sexual desire disorder (HSDD) in nondepressed women." *Journal of Sex and Marital Therapy*. (2001): 27, 303–316.

Seybold, V. S., J. W. Miller, and P. R. Lewis. "Investigation of a dopaminergic mechanism for regulating oxytocin release." *Journal of Pharmacology and Experimental Therapeutics*. (1978): 207, 605–610.

Shah, Y. "America's 'longest-married' couple wants to give you love advice." *Huffington Post*, 2/10/2016. http://www.huffingtonpost.com/entry/longest-married-couple-will-answer-your-questions-about-love_us_56bb4e72e4b0b 40245c4c0a3.

Shapiro, L. E., and T. R. Insel. "Oxytocin receptor distribution reflects social organization in monogamous and polygamous voles." *Annals of the New York Academy of Sciences*. (1992): 652: 448–451.

Shaver, P., J. Schwartz, D. Kirson, and C. O'Connor. "Emotion knowledge: Further exploration of a prototype approach." *Journal of Personality and Social Psychology*. (1987): 52, 1061–1086.

Shaver, P. R., H. J. Morgan, and S. Wu. "Is love a "basic" emotion?" *Personal Relationships*. (1996): 3, 81–96.

Shen, Q., et al. "To Cheat or Not To Cheat: Tryptophan Hydroxylase 2 SNP Variants Contribute to Dishonest Behavior." *Frontiers in Behavioral Neuroscience*. (May 2, 2016): 10: 82.

Sherwin, B. B. "Sex hormones and psychological functioning in postmenopausal women." *Experimental Gerontology*. (1994): 29, 423–430.

Small, D. M., R. J. Zatorre, A. Dagher, A. C. Evans, and M. Jones-Gotman.

"Changes in brain activity related to eating chocolate: From pleasure to aversion." *Brain*. (2001): 124, 1720–1733.

Smeltzer, M. D., J. T. Curtis, B. J. Aragona, and Z. Wang. "Dopamine, oxytocin, and vasopressin receptor binding in the medial prefrontal cortex of monogamous and promiscuous voles." *Neuroscience Letters*. (2006): 394(2): 146–151.

Smith, K. E., E. C. Porges, G. J. Norman, J. J. Connelly, and J. Decety. "Oxytocin receptor gene variation predicts empathic concern and autonomic arousal while perceiving harm to others." *Social Neuroscience*. (February, 2014): 9(1): 1–9.

Sokoloff, L. "Energetics of functional activation in neural tissues." *Neurochemical Research*. (1999): 24, 321–329.

Staes, N., S. E. Koski, P. Helsen, E. Fransen, M. Eens, and J. M. Stevens. "Chimpanzee sociability is associated with vasopressin (AVPR1a) but not Oxytocin receptor gene (OXTR) variation." *Hormones and Behavior*. (September, 2015): 75: 84–90.

Striepens, N., et al. "Oxytocin facilitates protective responses to aversive social stimuli in males." *Proceedings of the National Academy of Sciences, USA*. (2012): 109(44): 18144–18149.

Striepens, N., K. M. Kendrick, W. Maier, and R. Hurlemann. "Prosocial effects of oxytocin and clinical evidence for its therapeutic potential." *Frontiers in Neuroendocrinology*. (2011): 32(4): 426–450.

Striepens, N., A. Matusch, K. M. Kendrick, Y. Mihov, D. Elmenhorst, B. Becker, M. Lang, H. H. Coenen, W. Maier, R. Hurlemann, A. Bauer. "Oxytocin enhances attractiveness of unfamiliar female faces independent of the dopamine reward system." *Psychoneuroendocrinology*. (January, 2014): 39: 74–87.

Succu, S., F. Sanna, C. Cocco, T. Melis, A. Boi, G. L. Ferri, et al. "Oxytocin induces penile erection when injected into the ventral tegmental area of male rats: Role of nitric oxide and cyclic GMP." *The European Journal of Neuroscience*. (2008): 28, 813–21.

Sunnafrank, M., and A. J. Ramirez. "At first sight: persistent relational effects of get-acquainted conversations." *Journal of Social and Personal Relationships*. (2004): 21, 361–379.

Swaab, D. F., L. J. Gooren, and M. A. Hofman. "Brain research, gender and sexual orientation." *Journal of Homosexuality*. (1995): 28(3–4):283–301.

Szezypka, M. S., Q. Y. Zhou, and R. D. Palmiter. "Dopamine-stimulated sexual behavior is testosterone dependent in mice." *Behavioral Neuroscience*. (1998): 112, 1229–1235.

Tabak, B. A., M. E. McCullough, A. Szeto, A. J. Mendez, and P. M. McCabe. "Oxytocin indexes relational distress following interpersonal harms in women." *Psychoneuroendocrinology*. (2010): 36, 115–122.

Taylor, S. E., S. Saphire-Bernstein, and T. E. Seeman. "Are plasma oxytocin in women and plasma vasopressin in men biomarkers of distressed pair-bond relationships?" *Psychological Science*. (2010): 21, 3–7.

Thackare, H., H. Nicholson, and K. Whittington. "Oxytocin—its role in male reproduction and new potential therapeutic uses." *Human Reproduction Update*. (2006): 12, 437–48.

Theodoridou, A., A. C. Rowe, I. S. Penton-Voak, and P. J. Rogers. "Oxytocin and social perception: Oxytocin increases perceived facial trustworthiness and attractiveness." *Hormones and Behavior*. (2009): 56(1): 128–132.

Ursu, S., V. A. Stenger, M. K. Shear, M. R. Jones, and C. S. Carter. "Overactive action monitoring in obsessive-compulsive disorder: Evidence from functional magnetic resonance imaging." *Psychological Science*. (2003): 14, 347–353.

Van Anders, S. M., K. L. Goldey, and P. X. Kuo. "The steroid/peptide theory of social bonds: integrating testosterone and peptide responses for classifying social behavioral contexts." *Psychoneuroendocrinology*. (2011): 36, 1265–1275.

Van de Kar, L. D., A. D. Levy, Q. Li, and M. S. Brownfield. "A comparison of the oxytocin and vasopressin responses to the 5-HT1A agonist and potential anxiolytic drug alnespirone (S-20499)." *Pharmacology Biochemistry and Behavior*. (1998): 60, 677–683.

Van Goozen, S., V. M. Wiegant, E. Endert, F. A. Helmond, N. E. Van de Poll. "Psychoendocrinological assessment of the menstrual cycle: The relationship between hormones, sexuality, and mood." *Archives of Sexual Behavior*. (1997): 26, 359–382.

Velanova, K., L. L. Jacoby, M. E. Wheeler, M. P. McAvoy, S. E. Petersen, and R. L. Buckner. "Functional-anatomic correlates of sustained and transient processing components engaged during controlled retrieval." *The Journal of Neuroscience*. (2003): 23, 8460–8470.

Vitalo, A., J. Fricchione, M. Casali, Y. Berdichevsky, E. A. Hoge, S. L. Rauch, et al. "Nest making and oxytocin comparably promote wound healing in isolation-reared rats." *PLoS One*. (2009): 4, 5523.

Vizi, E. S., and V. Volbekas. "Inhibition by dopamine of oxytocin release from isolated posterior lobe of the hypophysis of the rat: Disinhibitory effect of beta-endorphin/enkephalin." *Neuroendocrinology*. (1980): 31, 46–52.

Vul, E., C. Harris, P. Winkielman, and H. Pashle. "Puzzlingly High Correlations in fMRI Studies of Emotion, Personality, and Social Cognition (the paper formerly known as 'Voodoo Correlations in Social Neuroscience')." http://laplab. ucsd.edu/articles/In%20press%20version/Vul_etal_2008inpress.pdf.

Walum, H., et al. "Variation in the oxytocin receptor gene is associated with pair-bonding and social behavior." *Biological Psychiatry*. (2012): 71(5): 419–426.

Wang, Y., et al. "NeuroPep: A comprehensive resource of neuropeptides." *Database (Oxford)*. (April 29, 2015): 2015:bav038.

Wang, Z., D. Toloczko, L. J. Young, K. Moody, J. D. Newman, and T. R. Insel. "Vasopressin in the forebrain of common marmosets (Calithrix jacchus): studies with in situ hybridization, immunocytochemistry and receptor autoradiography." *Brain Research*. (1997): 768, 147–156.

Wang, Z., G. Yu, C. Cascio, Y. Liu, B. Gingrich, and T. R. Insel. "Dopamine D2 receptor-mediated regulation of partner preferences in female prairie voles (Microtus ochrogaster): a mechanism for pair-bonding?" *Behavioral Neuroscience.* (1999): 113, 602–611.

Wang, Z. X., C. F. Ferris, and G. J. De Vries. "The role of septal vasopressin innervation in paternal behavior in prairie voles (Microtus ochrogaster)." *Proceedings of the National Academy of Sciences, USA.* (1994): 91, 400–404.

Wedekind, C., and S. Furi. "Body odour preferences in men and women: Do they aim for specific MHC combinations or simply heterozygosity?" *Proceedings of the Royal Society of London.* (1997): V264, 1387.

Wedekind, C., T. Seebeck, F. Bettens, and A. Paepke. "MHC-independent Mate Preferences in Humans." *Proceedings of the Royal Society B: Biological Sciences.* (1995): 260: 245–249.

Weisman, O., R. Feldman, and A. Goldstein. "Parental and romantic attachment shape brain processing of infant cues." *Biological Psychology.* (2011): 89(3): 533–8.

Wenkstern, D., J. G. Pfaus, and H. C. Fibiger. "Dopamine transmission increases in the nucleus accumbens of male rats during their first exposure to sexually receptive female rats." *Brain Research.* (1993): 618, 41–46.

Wersinger, S. R., and E. F. Rissman. "Dopamine activates masculine sexual behavior independent of the estrogen receptor alpha." *The Journal of Neuroscience.* (2000): 20, 4248–4254.

West, C. H. K., A. N. Clancy, and R. P. Michael. "Enhanced responses of nucleus accumbens neurons in male rats to novel odors associated with sexually receptive females." *Brain Research.* (1992): 585, 49–55.

White, N. M., and N. Hiroi. "Preferential localization of self-stimulation sites in striosomes/patches in the rat striatum." *Proceedings of the National Academy of Sciences, USA.* (1998): 95, 6486–6491.

White-Traut, R., K. Watanabe, H. Pournajafi-Nazarloo, D. Schwertz, A. Bell, and C. S. Carter. "Detection of salivary oxytocin levels in lactating women." *Developmental Psychobiology.* (2009): 51, 367–373.

Williams, J. R., T. R. Insel, C. R. Harbaugh, and C. S. Carter. "Oxytocin administered centrally facilitates formation of a partner preference in female prairie voles (Microtus ochrogaster)." *Journal of Neuroendocrinology.* (1994): 6, 247–250.

Williams, S. M., and P. S. Goldman-Rakic. "Widespread origin of the primate mesofrontal dopamine system." *Cerebral Cortex.* (1998): 8, 321–345.

Winslow, J. T., N. Hastings, C. S. Carter, C. R. Harbaugh, and T. R. Insel. "A role for central vasopressin in pair-bonding in monogamous prairie voles." *Nature.* (1993): 365, 545–548.

Wise, R. A. "Neurobiology of addiction." *Current Opinion in Neurobiology.* (1996): 6, 243–251.

Wise, R. A., and D. C. Hoffman. "Localization of drug reward mechanisms by intracranial injections." *Synapse*. (1992): 10, 247–263.

Wotjak, C. T., J. Ganster, G. Kohl, F. Holsboer, R. Landgraf, and M. Engelmann. "Dissociated central and peripheral release of vasopressin, but not oxytocin, in response to repeated swim stress: new insights into the secretory capacities of peptidergic neurons." *Neuroscience*. (1998): 85, 1209–1222.

Yadin, E., and E. Thomas. "Stimulation of the lateral septum attenuates immobilization-induced stress ulcers." *Physiological Behavior*. (1996): 59, 883–886.

Young, K. A., K. L. Gobrogge, Y. Liu, and Z. Wang. "The neurobiology of pair bonding: Insights from a socially monogamous rodent." *Frontiers in Neuroendocrinology*. (2011): 329(1): 53–69.

Young, L. "Being human: Love: Neuroscience reveals all." *Nature*. (2009): 457, 148.

Young, L. J., M. M. Lim, B. Gingrich, and T. R. Insel. "Cellular mechanisms of social attachment." *Hormones and Behavior*. (2001): 40, 133–138.

Young, L. J., Z. Wang, and T. R. Insel. "Neuroendocrine bases of monogamy." *Trends in Neurosciences*. (1998): 21, 71–75.

Young, L. J., J. T. Winslow, R. Nilsen, and T. R. Insel. "Species differences in V1a receptor gene expression in monogamous and nonmonogamous voles: Behavioral consequences." *Behavioral Neuroscience*. (1997): 111, 599–605.

Young, L. J. "Oxytocin and vasopressin receptors and species-typical social behaviors." *Hormones and Behavior*. (1999): 36, 212–221.

Zak, P., A. Stanton, and S. Ahmadi. "Oxytocin increases generosity in humans." *PLoS One*. (2007): 2, 1128.

Zhang, Y. M., et al. "Activation and blockade of prelimbic 5-HT6 receptors produce different effects on depressive-like behaviors in unilateral 6-hydroxydopamine-induced Parkinson's rats." *Neuropharmacology*. (July 14, 2016):110(pt. A): 25–36.

Zhaoping, L., et al. "Serotonin Reduces the Hyperpolarization-Activated Current (IN) in Ventral Tegmental Area Dopamine Neurons: Involvement of 5-HT2 Receptors and Protein Kinase C." *Journal of Neurophysiology*. (November, 2003): 90(5): 3201–12.

# ABOUT THE AUTHOR

Fred Nour was born in Cairo, Egypt in the 1950s, the son of teachers who were both Coptic Christians. (Copts are descendants of the Pharaohs, and the Coptic language of today is a variation of the ancient Egyptian hieroglyphics.)

In his senior medical school year at Egypt's Cairo University, the Muslim Brotherhood movement started to become more powerful and popular. Nour felt his future in the country as a minority was threatened. After graduation near the top of his class, he began planning to move to the United States. The country's modern advanced medicine and belief that success in the United States is regardless of race, color, religion, or wealth made him certain he would succeed or fail in the United States based solely on his abilities.

The US embassy in Cairo told him if he passed a test, the "Educational Commission on Foreign Medical Graduates," they would give him an application to complete. Egypt wasn't listed as an examination site, so he chose London, which he'd visited before. After numerous failed attempts, he succeeded in getting an exit visa from Egypt, but at that time, he could only leave Cairo with 110 English pounds. Thanks to a person in London who wanted to send money to his family in Egypt, he ended up in London with 310 English pounds.

He arrived in London four days before his examination, in the first week of July 1977, and found a rental room. It would be the end of September before he could make application at the American embassy for the trip to the United States, and he spent the time in between focusing on improving his spoken English by watching TV and attempting to comprehend each and every word he heard.

Finally, the letter came in the mail, and, hallelujah, he passed on his first attempt! After a sleepless night, armed with his passport and the letter, he walked into the American embassy and presented both.

The US embassy employee told him, "Sorry, sir, we no longer accept this for physician immigration. Due to the end of the Vietnam War, we now have a glut of doctors in the United States. If you want to immigrate as a physician, there's another examination, a competitive examination, the Visa Qualifying Examination, which we call the VQE. We take a preset number of the doctors starting with the top scores and give the preset number of doctors immigration visas."

Nour wasn't bothered by this; he'd already been through the grueling competition of medical school and had passed the first test easily. But then the man said, "All this has just happened, so it will take time to set it up. Please check with us every six months, and we'll tell you when you can take it."

Shocked and disappointed, he took the Underground back to his room in Muswell Hill. On the train, he thought about his options—either go back to Egypt as a failure and be at the mercy of the Muslim Brotherhood, or persevere and keep fighting his way to America. The decision was clear: he would stay in London, practice there until the test was available, take it, pass it, and then go back to the embassy to apply again.

Arriving home, he told his landlady, a kindly, elderly Irishwoman named Trish, the news, and that he had to find a practice position in England. Two days later, she returned from an appointment with her GP bearing a piece of paper. On it were the words, "General Medical Council in London." Nour went there the next day.

Another examination was needed, and the next opening was six long weeks away. The 120 pounds left with him wouldn't sustain him until then. He asked if there was a way for him to stay at a local hospital until the examination. Luck was with him: the GMC had a "clinical observer" program, where he could stay at a hospital to observe the British doctors. This program wasn't available in London, but he gratefully took the list of hospitals that offered it.

Cheltenham General Hospital had a vacancy for one doctor, observing a Dr. Maines, in internal medicine. If accepted, Nour could stay in a room in the nurses' residence for 5 pounds per week, and eat for free at the doctors' dining room. He simply could not believe his good fortune when his request was approved.

The clinical observer position wasn't in his specialty, but he still gained valuable experience following Dr. Maines on his rounds every day, and Dr. Maines seemed to relish the chance to answer and also ask

Nour questions about the cases they saw together. Nour was equally as challenged in the evenings by Dr. Flowers, head of the hospital's Accident and Emergency Department. Nour's confidence in his medical knowledge grew each day.

On the day of the exam, Nour took the first coach from Cheltenham to London, and soon after the written test, he qualified to take the oral clinical examination thanks to his experience with Dr. Maines, in taking care of a case where hyperbaric oxygen was the most recent way to treat it. Even better, it turned out the examiner had trained with Dr. Maines and knew him well. He passed the oral exam, and would receive a letter with the result in three to five days.

The first thing he wanted to do when back at the hospital was to go to the doctors' lounge to eat. Two minutes after he arrived, Dr. Flowers sat next to him and asked him to show up in his office the next day, Friday, at eight a.m., "for a very important matter."

Friday at eight a.m., he was at Dr. Flowers's office, apprehensive. He needn't have been. Dr. Flowers found out that Nour had passed his exam, and said, "Congratulations, in about one hour you will start your first job in England."

A faxed copy of the results in hand, Nour visited administration to do the employment paperwork, and then walked to the A&E ward to start to see patients.

Doing well in this position quickly led to others, and to prove to the British that he was just as good as any of them, he decided to take two examinations: the LRCP (Licentiate of the Royal College of Physicians) and MRCS (Member of the Royal College of Surgeons). The examinations required two years of training in the United Kingdom, but by then he'd heard that the long-awaited VQE exam had been scheduled after he finished only one year of the UK training. He decided to finish the two years of training in the UK first and then take the American VQE exam the second year, hopeful that turning down the first date wouldn't end his chance of going to the United States. He passed the LRCP and MRCS, and became licensed as a "Full Permanent Registered Physician" on the British register of qualified physicians.

Of just over seven thousand physicians taking the VQE examination that year, US immigration would only accept the top three hundred. He still dreamed of immigrating to America, but numbers like that didn't worry him anymore; if he failed, he would happily stay and practice in the UK.

He took the VQE examination. The result came in the mail. He qualified for a visa.

Armed with this letter and his passport, he made the by then familiar trip to the American embassy. Interestingly, he was met by the same employee as before—and bearing similar news. "Sorry, Dr. Nour, this year they added a new requirement to even apply: a Labor Certificate in addition to the VQE result."

Fighting the urge to chuckle, Nour replied, "That's fine; how do I get this Labor Certificate?"

"You have to get a job in the USA. It has to be advertised in a professional journal for doctors." Not only that, but the ad had to list a PO Box address and require that all applicants reply that way. "Replies to this box get forwarded to the Labor Department," he explained. "If someone who's a legal US resident applies, he gets the job, and you don't qualify. If nobody applies for ninety days, the Labor Department will issue you the Labor Certificate, certifying that no equally qualified US legal resident is available to fill the job. With the VQE result and the Labor Certificate, you can apply for an immigration visa."

Although there was a series of hoops to jump through this time, Nour remained positive. He realized he had to somehow get closer to the United States in order to get interviews and then hopefully a job offer. Canada looked likely. But similar to the United States, he needed a job offer there to get this registration.

He scoured the Canadian and British medical journals for job vacancies and found an ad for a general practitioner in a small town in Saskatchewan called Kincaid. They'd retained a professional consultant to help with this. Nour contacted him. The consultant arranged everything, from the flight from London to a bus to Saskatoon for the medical boards to an appointment with the registrar there. After arriving, he discovered Kincaid's population was three hundred. Three hundred people, that was. He later discovered that most of the populace were farmers living on huge farms. He started work as Kincaid's sole GP. Now he could survive while applying for jobs in the United States.

The applications didn't always go his way. He was offered a job in McKeesport, Pennsylvania, but first, the job must be advertised as required by the Labor Department. An Indian doctor, whose immigration was approved because of his brother being a US citizen, got that job.

Another job in Jacksonville, Florida was taken by a Latin American applicant who was married to an American woman.

The third job offer came from New Orleans, Louisiana, a one-year assignment to an LSU (Louisiana State University) program. This time, no US citizen applied for the entire ninety days! He qualified to get an immigration visa now—but he was told he still had to wait six months, this time so the Labor Department employee in charge could sign the Labor Certificate.

Deciding he was finished with the hoop-jumping, eager to finally begin a career practice, Nour discovered the famed value of American lawyers. He hired an immigration lawyer to help him, and the required medical exams, a multitude of forms, criminal background checks—all of it suddenly moved smoothly.

His lawyer called him to drive down from Saskatchewan, Canada to the New Orleans federal building. Together they met the government immigration lawyer inside to review the papers. In just fifteen minutes, he heard words he'd been hoping to hear for a long time: "Congratulations, you are now a legal permanent resident in the USA." He couldn't resist the tears coming down his cheeks.

The government immigration lawyer said, "I'm sorry, Doctor, I know we make it hell for you to come here, but we have to carefully follow all the procedures. You can now walk to Charity Hospital and start working today."

Nour looked at him, startled. "But I don't have any papers to prove that I can work legally."

"No problem, Doctor, we'll stamp your passport saying, 'Employment is authorized.'"

By the time the next hurdle appeared, Nour was well aware that finding professional success didn't mean that no hurdles were left for him in life.

All residency training starts on July first. Nour had completed his internship late, since he started late due to the immigration delay. He had to wait six months to begin his residency, so to fill in the time gap he got a temporary job in Chicago as an emergency room physician on Chicago's South Side. He discovered he really liked Chicago, a lot.

When he completed his internship at LSU New Orleans, he sought a residency position in neurology, his chosen specialty. He applied to five programs in the Southeast, and all five accepted him. He ended up at the

Baylor College of Medicine in Houston, Texas, one of the top 10 in the nation. His neurology residency was finished in 1986.

But he still liked Chicago, a lot. After his training, he elected to go back to Chicago to practice neurology in a suburban setting. Of the two hospitals he liked the most, he chose Central DuPage Hospital in west suburban Chicago. He didn't know one single physician there. He didn't know one single person in that area, but he had confidence that after all the heartaches, he could compete with anybody and beat any obstacle.

He spent the first three years teaching neurology part-time at the University of Illinois and lived by a lake in suburban Chicago. The lake had a small island and was surrounded by trees, and his house was close to the water, perhaps fifteen to twenty feet from the shoreline. When he bought the house, it had a pair of Canada geese, which he found an interesting addition to living beside a lake. Gradually over the years, these two geese multiplied to a hundred or two! He started to get a cough every spring and fall. The specialists he consulted thought it was asthma. Gradually he developed fevers and chills, symptoms not typical of asthma. After visiting a few large medical centers with no diagnosis, he felt he had to diagnose it himself.

A few years of research, and he made the connection, and diagnosed himself with hypersensitivity pneumonitis caused by the Canada geese exposure. This is an allergic pneumonia, so it has the symptoms of pneumonia but without any infection. Wanting to make sure his diagnosis was the right one after being misdiagnosed before, he went to the nation's top expert in that disease at Northwest University in Chicago. There are no commercially available tests for this, so the diagnosis was confirmed by specialized laboratory tests custom made for him. His case was published in 2000, under the title, "Hypersensitivity pneumonitis resulting from community exposure to Canada goose droppings: when an external environmental antigen becomes an indoor environmental antigen," in the medical journal *Annals of Allergy, Asthma and Immunology*.

There is no treatment for this disease except to avoid exposure to the cause, which in Nour's case was the Canada geese droppings. This meant he had to move away from the little house by the lake. He moved to another house in Chicago, in a wooded area, and relocated his office. However, with the Chicago area being heavily populated with Canada geese by then, he couldn't totally avoid exposure to their droppings.

After a few more years fighting with this disease, he relocated to

Indiana in 2007, seeing that the geese population there was smaller. In a few years the geese population expanded further, and he kept getting sick. In 2011 he moved to Southern California, where the geese population is smaller due to the lack of grass and freshwater lakes. He hopes this will be his last move.

Dr. Nour holds two board certifications from the American Board of Psychiatry and Neurology. He was named as one of the "Top Chicago Physicians" in 2003, and as one of "America's Top Physicians" in 2005, 2006, 2009, and 2010. He was named one of the "Top Doctors in Indianapolis" in 2011.

He enjoys portrait oil painting, sailing, traveling, and learning about other cultures. He is an avid opera fan and, understandably, prefers to admire geese from afar.

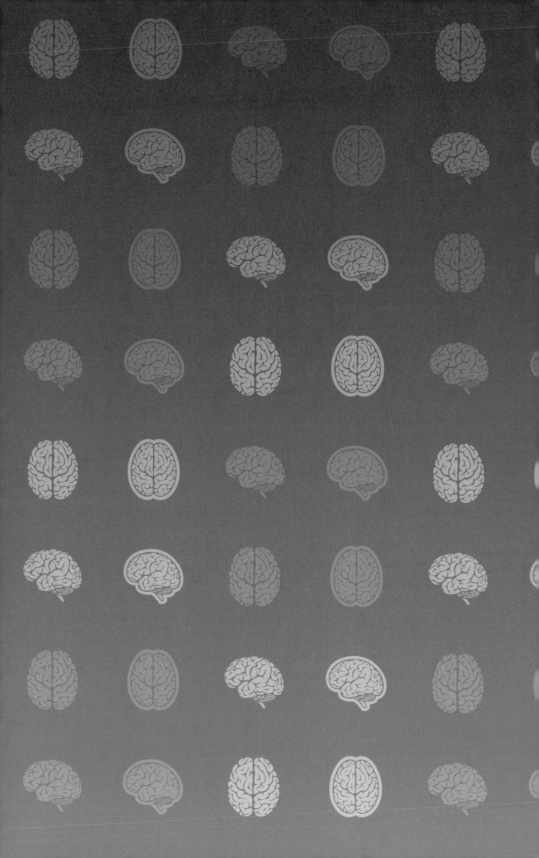

# CREDITS / COPYRIGHT

## Figures

Ancient Egyptian vase. ©Tatty.

Inanna and Dumuzi. Public domain.

Basic brain parts. Illustration by author. ©Fred Nour.

Frog's brain. ©2007 Thomas J. Herbert.

Bird's brain. Adapted from Jarvis, E. D., et. al. "Global view of the functional molecular organization of the avian cerebrum: mirror images and functional columns." Journal of Comparative Neurology. 521(16), 2013. John Wiley & Sons.

Smell and attraction. Adobe stock photo. ©nastia1983.

Human brain. Adobe stock photo. ©decade3d.

Is love in the heart or the brain? ©Sellingpix / Dreamstime.com.

Sex and the brain. ©freshidea.

My daughter's wedding plan. Provided by author's daughter

Woman holding her golden egg. ©Sergey Nivens.

Peacock eyespots. ©Zonda.

Peacock. ©Ievgen Melamud.

Cell communication model. Images: ©aey, ©Leo Blanchette. Art: ©Fred Nour.

Basal ganglia, dopamine networks in Parkinson's disease. ©Charles Michael Gibson.

Basic sensory nerves. Author artwork. ©Fred Nour.

Hoarding. Source: Wikimedia / Grap.

Swinging together. ©tatoman.

Carmen and Don José. Magdalena Kožená and Jonas Kaufmann at the Salzburg Festival 2012. Photo by Luigi Caputo / Wikipedia.

Bette Davis & Leslie Howard in *Of Human Bondage*. Public domain.

Divorce graph: USA divorces by duration of marriage, 1990. US

Department of Health and Human Services, Center for Disease Control, National Center for Health Statistics: "Advance Report of Final Divorce Statistics 1989–1990."

A vole. ©David Peskens / Dreamstime.com.

Oxytocin is needed throughout our life cycle. Source: "Oxytocin: The great facilitator of life." Heon-Jin Lee, Abbe H. Macbeth, Jerome H. Pagani, W. Scott Young 3rd. *Progress in Neurobiology*, Volume 88, Issue 2, June 2009, Pages 127–151. Elsevier.

This is the True Love we should all seek. Public domain.

Limbic brain centers, side view. Source: Website, "The Pixelated Brain" by Dana C. Brooks, MD. www.pixelatedbrain.com. ©2011. Used by permission of Dana C. Brooks, MD.

Limbic brain centers, top view. Source: Website, "The Pixelated Brain" by Dana C. Brooks, MD. www.pixelatedbrain.com. ©2011. Used by permission of Dana C. Brooks, MD.

Hypothalamic nuclei. Source: Public share.

EEG, provided by author. ©Fred Nour.

Side view of MRI of the brain. Provided by author. ©Fred Nour

Top view of MRI of the brain. Provided by author. ©Fred Nour

Susceptibility MRI. Provided by author. ©Fred Nour

MRS. Public domain

fMRI. This image purportedly shows brain reaction to looking at faces versus buildings. US Department of Health and Human Services, National Institute of Mental Health.

TMS. Used with permission of Mayo Foundation for Medical Education and Research, all rights reserved.

Vagal nerve stimulation. ©Cyberonics.

DTI. Provided by author. ©Fred Nour

MRA. Provided by author. ©Fred Nour

## Tables

Monoamines overview. By author. ©Fred Nour.

Cell communication names (by author with diagrams). ©Fred Nour, ©aey, and ©Leo Blanchette.

Vole comparison. By author. ©Fred Nour.

Summary of brain chemicals involved in love. By author. ©Fred Nour.

Outline of hypothalamic centers and their functions. By author. ©Fred Nour.

## Songs & Poems

**Song:** "A New Day Has Come." Words and Music by Aldo Nova Caporuscio and Stephan Moccio. Copyright ©2002 BMG Gold Songs, Viral Records, and Sing Little Penguin. All rights for BMG Gold Songs and Viral Records administered by BMG Rights Management (US) LLC. All rights for Sing Little Penguin administered by Songs of Universal, Inc. All rights reserved. Used by permission. Reprinted by permission of Hal Leonard LLC.

**Song:** "Because You Loved Me" (theme from the film *Up Close and Personal*). Words and Music by Diane Warren. ©1996 Realsongs (ASCAP) and Touchstone Pictures Songs & Music, Inc. (ASCAP). All rights reserved. Used by permission of Hal Leonard LLC & Alfred Music.

**Song:** "How Can I Not Love You." Words and Music by George Fenton, Kenneth "Babyface" Edmonds, and Robert Kraft. Copyright ©1999 Fox Film Music Corp., Sony/ATV Songs LLC, and ECAF Music. All rights on behalf of Sony/ATV Songs LLC and ECAF Music administered by Sony/ATV Music Publishing, 424 Church Street, Suite 1200, Nashville, TN 37219. All rights reserved. Used by permission. Reprinted by permission of Hal Leonard LLC.

**Song:** "Maria" (from *West Side Story*) by Leonard Bernstein, lyrics by Stephen Sondheim. Copyright ©1956, 1957, 1958, 1959 by Amberson Holdings LLC and Stephen Sondheim. Copyright renewed, Leonard Bernstein Music Publishing Company LLC, Publisher. Boosey & Hawkes, Agent for Rental. International copyright secured. Reprinted by permission.

**Song:** "My Heart Will Go On" (Love Theme from *Titanic*), from the Paramount and Twentieth Century Fox Motion Picture *Titanic*. Music by James Horner. Lyric by Will Jennings. Copyright ©1997 Sony/ATV Harmony, Sony/ATV Melody, TCF Music Publishing, Inc., Fox Film Music Corporation, and Blue Sky Rider Songs. All rights on behalf of Sony/ATV Harmony and Sony/ATV Melody administered by Sony/ATV Music

# INDEX

Note: an *f* indicates a figure; a *t* a table.

# NOTES

# NOTES

"With more than 30 years of experience as a neurologist and a researcher, I can say without hesitation that True Love is the most comprehensive and effective life skills book I have ever seen. If you are interested in understanding the reality of love, I strongly recommend this book for you. Simple, enchanting and educational yet has the power to inspire and transform attitudes and behaviors. From the outset, readers are encouraged to understand facts and apply them directly to their own lives and in doing so can grasp seemingly complex medical concepts. The language spoken allows any individual to integrate learning and develop an enquiring mind with great self-reflection. This sets the scene for them to become in charge of their own love lives with the potential to achieve true everlasting love."

—Richard Dubinsky, M.D., MPH.

*Professor of Neurology, Kansas City*
*Member, Quality Standards subcommittee of the America Academy of Neurology*
*Member, Technology and Therapeutics committee of the America Academy of Neurology*
*Chairman, Practice Improvement subcommittee of the American Academy of Neurology*
*Vice-chairman, Quality Measures Reporting subcommittee of the American Academy of Neurology*
*Consulting Neurologist at Kansas City Zoological Gardens*

"This book is beyond inspiring. A heartfelt, wise, scientific, honest and entertaining book about our deepest emotion: love. Enormously helpful to all of us who want to understand our love-lives. This great book, true love, is a treasure that I will share with many of my personal and professional friends."

—John Ellis, M.D.

*Neurologist, Amarillo, Texas*

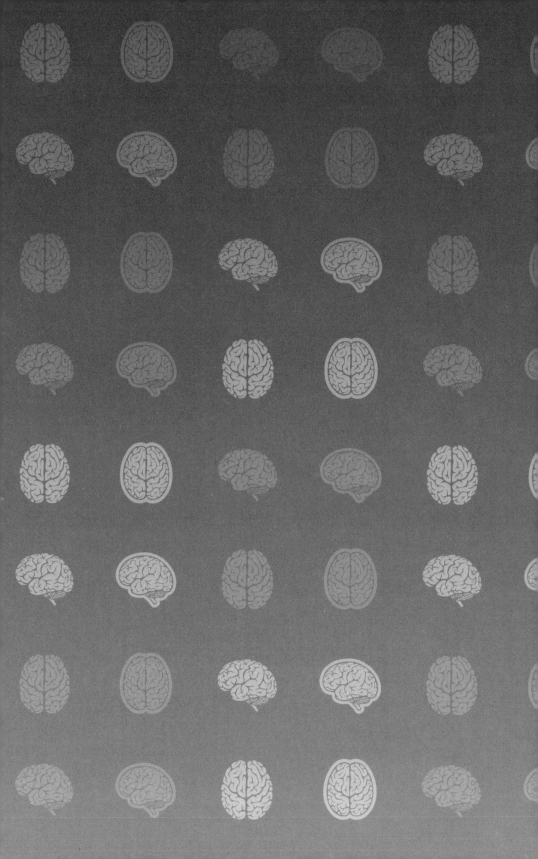